E-attachment and Online Communication

This book examines the use of modern technologies in clinical psychological practice. It considers how we define attachment in an age where changes in technology and the COVID-19 pandemic have increased the prevalence of online contact in the process of diagnosis and psychological treatment.

Based on an attachment paradigm that is relatively unexplored, the book outlines how modern online contact influences mental health and development, along with the therapeutic relationship between client and professional. It discusses people's relationships with new technologies, how relationships can be established using these technologies, and how these technologies affect professional relationships between psychologists and their clients, which they define as e-attachment. In the context of new technologies, the book draws on neurobiology and clinical psychology to consider mental health, social functioning, and emotional regulation.

Presenting both theory and examples from case studies, this cutting-edge book will be of great interest to researchers, academics, and post-graduate students in the fields of clinical psychology, psychotherapy, and mental health. Those also carrying out research into digital and online learning within the field of mental health will also benefit from this text.

Katarzyna Sitnik–Warchulska is Clinical Psychologist, Child and Adolescent Psychotherapist and Assistant Professor at the Institute of Applied Psychology, Jagiellonian University, Poland.

Bernadetta Izydorczyk is Clinical Psychologist, Psychotherapist and Supervisor of Psychotherapy, and Associate Professor at the Institute of Psychology, Jagiellonian University, Poland.

Zbigniew Wajda is Clinical Psychologist, Psychotherapist and Assistant Professor at the Institute of Applied Psychology, Jagiellonian University, Poland.

Explorations in Mental Health

Applications of a Psychospiritual Model in the Helping Professions
Principles of InnerView Guidance
Cedric Speyer and John Yaphe

Effective Group Therapies for Young Adults Affected by Cancer
Using Support Groups in Clinical Settings in the United States
Sarah F. Kurker

Fostering Resilience Before, During, and After Experiences of Trauma
Insights to Inform Practice Across the Lifetime
Edited by Buuma Maisha, Stephanie Massicotte and Melanie Morin

Hip-Hop and Spoken Word Therapy in School Counseling
Developing Culturally Responsive Approaches
Ian Levy

Compassionate Love in Intimate Relationship
The Integration Process of Sexual Mass Trauma, Racism, and Resilience
Josiane M. Apollon

Trauma and its Impacts on Temporal Experience
New Perspectives from Phenomenology and Psychoanalysis
Selene Mezzalira

Self and Identity
An Exploration of the Development, Constitution and Breakdown of Human Selfhood
Matthew Tieu

For more information about this series, please visit www.routledge.com/Explorations-in-Mental-Health/book-series/EXMH

E-attachment and Online Communication

The Changing Context of the Clinical Diagnosis and Psychological Treatment

Katarzyna Sitnik-Warchulska,
Bernadetta Izydorczyk, and
Zbigniew Wajda

Routledge
Taylor & Francis Group

LONDON AND NEW YORK

First published 2023
by Routledge
4 Park Square, Milton Park, Abingdon, Oxon OX14 4RN

and by Routledge
605 Third Avenue, New York, NY 10158

Routledge is an imprint of the Taylor & Francis Group, an informa business

British Library Cataloguing-in-Publication Data
A catalogue record for this book is available from the British Library

Library of Congress Cataloging-in-Publication Data
A catalog record has been requested for this book

ISBN: 978-1-032-11686-0 (hbk)
ISBN: 978-1-032-11687-7 (pbk)
ISBN: 978-1-003-22104-3 (ebk)

DOI: 10.4324/9781003221043

Typeset in Bembo
by MPS Limited, Dehradun

We would like to thank our lovedones for presence and inspiration

The translation and open access license fee of the publication were funded by the Priority Research Area Society of the Future under the program "Excellence Initiative – Research University" at the Jagiellonian University in Krakow.

Contents

Introduction

At the end of the 20th century, a breakthrough took place that permanently changed human functioning. Ubiquitous technology has opened up new possibilities for communication and contact with people from all over the world. It also posed a man and his Self to a number of questions about the limits of his functioning and the nature of humanity. The moment of writing this book coincided with the time when generations brought up in hybrid reality enter adult life, building their identity both in the real and virtual world. These are the times when technology is also increasingly present in the process of diagnosis and treatment of patients. Internet applications, virtual reality (VR) glasses, robots with social functions are a reality that is already widely used in the process of helping and psychotherapy at the time of writing this book. The use of avatars or the presence of humanoid robots in the healing process is no longer an image known from Sci-Fi literature and it becomes an announcement of scientists about the near future. This process of entering the virtual world into the world of direct relationships was further strengthened by the COVID-19 pandemic. Using the advances of technology has, in fact, become the norm around the world. At the same time, it is also the moment when mainly people whose lives experience a technological breakthrough in the course of their development write about the possibilities and consequences of combining real and virtual reality. After all, it is a time of discussion and asking open questions about whether and how to translate the bond and social touch to the virtual world, what consequences this has for shaping attachment, and consequently for symptoms of psychopathology, diagnosis and treatment with the use of technology embedded in the online world.

This book is the effect of the authors' reflection on the phenomenon, review of research and clinical observations regarding the use of modern technologies in clinical psychological practice, with particular emphasis on attachment. The authors focus on explaining how modern online contact may have an influence on bonds, in consequence, on mental health and development, symptoms progress and the therapeutic diagnostic relationship between the client and the professional.

DOI: 10.4324/9781003221043-1

The first chapter describes the broad context of human development, mental and social functioning in the context of new technologies. It discussed the contemporary psychological and socio-cultural context of changes in development, including impacts of technology use on communication skills, self-development and forming personality. It discusses "if" and "how" behavioral, emotional and social generations growing up during significant overlapping changes – technology development and pandemics. It discusses the issues of mediated social touch and the area of research on the digital touch phenomenon. The last part of the chapter focuses on the discussion on the hybrid of functioning and psychosocial development of modern man in the context of the boundaries between the real (offline) and virtual (online) world.

Chapter 2 focuses on the subject of attachment in the age of digital human functioning. It describes the changes in defining and looking at this phenomenon, in theoretical, research and clinical terms. It discusses the cultural-attachment construct. Is the virtual world only an extension of the attachment pattern formed in direct physical contact with loved ones? Doesn't the hybrid reality invite contemporary generations to take a different view of the attachment nature? Is it not legitimate to discuss attachment in the context of E-attachment? These are the questions that are discussed in this chapter. The E-attachment model proposed in it is a proposal to capture the complexity of factors determining attachment, and at the same time to take into account its new dimension, shaped in the dynamic offline-online reality.

Chapter 3 presents issues related to attachment, interpersonal relations (including psychologist–client) and modern technologies from the perspective of neuroscience. It discusses the neuronal and physiological correlates of attachment in the context of human-to-human contact as well as online interaction. The review of positions on neurobiology and attachment became the starting point for analyzes focused on social neuroscience, neural and physiological forms of bonding and online therapeutic relationships, the roles of the brain components in the process of creating relationships in the online environment. Does the therapeutic relationship via the Internet change the functioning of the brain? The last part of Chapter 3 is devoted to this key issue.

Chapter 4 highlights the links between new technologies and broadly understood mental health using attachment theory. The chapter compares the understanding of attachment disorders and the tradition of thinking about psychopathology with a contemporary perspective, capturing the key importance of modern ICT for human development. The influence of modern technologies on shaping mental disorders such as anxiety disorders, depression, personality disorders, eating disorders, addictions and psychological crises was discussed. The second part of the chapter is focused on the analysis of relatively new clinical phenomena related to the use of modern technologies, such as harmful use of the Internet, video games, streaming platforms or cyberbullying.

Chapter 5 describes contemporary trends in diagnosis and psychological treatment using new technologies (video training, online platforms, social media, mobile applications, etc.). It presents selected treatment programs using modern technologies. In response to the need for an interdisciplinary diagnosis and therapy adapted to the requirements of the modern world, it presents research on the effectiveness of counseling and treatment with the use of online and ICT technology. The last part of the chapter presents recommendations for diagnostic and therapeutic management in the psychosocial model, with the use of modern technological tools (such as internet platforms, applications, video training, tele-advice and e-advice).

Chapter 6, the last one, presents the specificity of dilemmas and challenges facing the psychologist nowadays, in the age of ubiquitous new technologies especially trying to establish professional relationships and attachments using this new technology (e-attachment). COVID-19 pandemic widespread on a huge scale the need to use new technologies during diagnostic and therapeutic contact online to ensure psychological help and maintain the mental balance of people with emotional difficulties. The chapter presents and analyzes the cases from the authors' own practice. They are treated as a starting point for the formulation of questions about the effectiveness of online diagnosis and therapy, the need for a separate theoretical paradigm to conceptualize the diagnostic and therapeutic relationship taking place in a hybrid or virtual reality, and finally questions about the limitations and ethical issues of this type of contact. The future will bring an answer to the question: does building relationships based on modern technologies be a chance for diagnosis and psychological help or a threat to their effectiveness?

It is worth noting that when writing this monograph, we were not accompanied by the ambition to resolve the questions and dilemmas presented in it related to shaping attachment in the new reality, also based on functioning in the virtual world. Assuming, however, that the hybrid world is more than a simple offline plus online connection, we are left with the question of whether the nature of attachment itself has changed? Is there a need for a new understanding of this phenomenon? Are the current theories and paradigms used in this area in diagnostic and therapeutic thinking sufficient? We invite you to consider and look for a new perspective on attachment and online communication.

Katarzyna Sitnik-Warchulska, Bernadetta Izydorczyk, Zbigniew Wajda

Chapter 1

Human development changes in the modern world

Chapter overview

The following chapter is devoted to considerations on the changes that man has undergone, in the context of development, in the era of technology and digitization. It assumes that man develops in interaction with the environment and that his development trajectory is the result of the action of the entire system of biological, personality, socio-cultural and environmental factors. Factors which, depending on the context, are risk factors or protective factors. The first part of the chapter deals with the issue of the impact of computerization of life and information and communication technology on human nature, their importance in the process of developmental changes throughout life, as a consequence of the changes that human psychosocial functioning has undergone. Reference was made to the discussion in the scientific and social space about the need to separate a new generation – the digital generation. It also discusses how the behavioral, emotional and social functioning of the growing up has changed during significant overlapping changes – the technology development and pandemics. The second part of the chapter deals in detail with the issue of social touch, as it is crucial for human development. The phenomenon of mediated social touch with the use of modern digital technologies was discussed, as well as the area of reflection on the phenomenon of digital touch. The chapter is an invitation to a discussion about the hybrid form of functioning and development of modern man and the boundaries in the combined offline world (direct physical contacts) and the online world (virtual reality).

Contemporary understanding of development

The changes that a person undergoes throughout his life arouses constant interest in research and clinical communities. Decades of reflection on what is developmental and what is not reflected in popular theoretical models of mental development. The conviction that normative development is based on facing the phases of life that follow in a specific sequence already connects the

DOI: 10.4324/9781003221043-2

classic theories of Freud, Erikson, Kohlberg and Piaget (Green and Piel, 2016). Consequently, clinical psychological diagnosis for many years focused on the aspect of differentiating the norm from psychopathology (nosological diagnosis). On the other hand, therapeutic interactions were mainly aimed at reducing symptoms.

Over time, however, it turned out that such a reductionist approach was insufficient. The ideas of life-span developmental psychology, popularized in the second half of the 20th century, indicated the need to perceive a human being as an individual susceptible to a varying degree to the modification of mental functions (intraindividual plasticists), developing in a multidimensional way until the end of life (Baltes, 1987). Moreover, it began to be emphasized that the changes that a person goes through in the course of his life are based on both progress and regression. Models related to positive youth development have emerged, emphasizing each young person's ability to grow and develop (Lerner et al., 2015a). Above all, it was noted that a person is embedded in a biological and personality context as well as a historical and cultural context (Lerner et al., 2015b).

These ideas are developed especially in recent years. At present, it is undisputed that a person develops in mutual interaction with the environment (ideas of Relational developmental systems RDS) (Lerner et al., 2015b). Consequently, understanding modern man seems impossible without taking into account his fundamental personal qualities, status, value system, characteristics of the context in which he lives and his ability to adapt, and at the same time influence on the environment in which he lives. Each of these factors may not only be protective but also, under certain conditions, constitute a risk factor for the development of maladaptive behavior. In the clinical context, it is therefore important to assume that the individual trajectory of human development, personality, identity and psychopathological symptoms is both consistency and change (Wilson and Olino, 2021). Resources as well as dysfunctions are therefore not "given". They reveal themselves in a mutual, responsive relationship with the environment. So far, the value of physical contact as a driving force for development has been emphasized mainly. Body contact, touch, responsive and social touch-oriented physical presence, known as social touch, are considered the basis for the development of communication skills, attachment, and emotional and cognitive regulation from the first days of life (Cascio et al., 2019; Norholt, 2020).

Hybrid man

In the age of technology and global digitization, contact with other people is more and more often done through electronic media. The Internet, remote forms of study and work, telephone applications, communication using emoticons or via social media are not trends anymore, but permanent elements of human life. Information and communication technology (ICT) is increasingly recognized and used in all areas of life, including education, diagnosis, and treatment (Galapathy et al., 2017). Portable Electronic Devices (PEDs) have become an extension of our Self. This is especially true of the generations of children and adolescents who are currently growing up. Influencer, YouTuber, vlogger, etc. are terms that quickly took root in the colloquial language of teenagers. The famous question "Who do you want to become when you grow up" asked in the 2019 online survey by Harris Poll/ LEGO® touched the public. It drew the world's attention to the fact that, in the opinion of adolescent children, YouTuber/vlogger is not only a profession but also a profession at the top of the list of the most desirable professions of the future in the surveyed population of children from the UK and the USA. The image of a teenager immersed in a telephone conversation, learning online and spending time mainly in virtual reality became permanent in the times of the pandemic. It is accompanied by the experience of accessibility, the removal of barriers in movement, exchange of thoughts and goods, and at the same time the experience of greater isolation and less direct contact with other people. This raises the question of the participation and role of ICT in shaping the path of development of modern generations, including emotional and interpersonal competences.

For the generation of people born and growing up in the period of intensive technological progress, computerization and digitization of everyday life, it is used to say Digital Generation or E-generation. These terms began to appear in scientific and popular science publications at the turn of the 21st century (Buckingham, 2006; Brillet et al., 2011). They partially referred to the descriptions of Millennials, Generation Y or Generation Z. The concepts of E-generation or digital-generation do not, however, serve to fully define the generation of people born in the second half of the 1990s and later. They are rather slogans symbolizing growth and development in the company of digital technology. The ongoing discussions on the legitimacy of using this type of concept show how important this change is.

Buckingham (2006) suggests that the inclusion of digital technology in life in the sense that it refers to a generational change that it concerns the social, widespread anxiety about the occurrence of irreversible change. In this sense, the functioning of information and communication technology and digital media can be treated as a breakthrough close to the great crises. But is this the same crisis for everyone? Can you talk about a distinct, generation-different person?

It seems that technological progress is primarily a change for those who, for a certain part of their lives, developed without access to media, telecommunications and IT devices or had limited access to them. In turn, for those who were born in the world of universal digitization, technology and audiovisual equipment are part of everyday life. Children and adolescents born in the 21st century grow in line with technological advances. Internet, digital readers, mobile phones, video games, the so-called wearable digital gadgets are a constant element of the social functioning of today's adolescent children and adolescents (Suresh and Glenda, 2018; Sivalingam and Subbaiyan, 2018). In some way, messengers, short digital messages and chats are a form of communication and social communication that they commonly use. Internet applications have become a permanent part of the education and development process. In the network, young people often find answers to the questions that bother them about identity, sexuality and social trends. They easily use modern ICT achievements to communicate with the world, expand the limits of their social functioning, as well as education. The world of communication technologies and the internet is attractive because what it offers is more profitable than physical reality and available in terms of time or money (Ersoy, 2019). A systematic review by Suresh and Glenda (2018) indicates that contemporary students see digital technology as a source of success. Digital technology has permanently changed the face of upbringing and education. Undoubtedly, access to knowledge can be a resource that increases the chances of developing one's competences. Suresh and Glenda (2018) emphasize that for the effective use of digital technology tools, it is important to conduct research on the impact of online culture on well-being, especially in the group of children and adolescents who have contact with ICT from an early age. It seems particularly important to trace the development trajectories of people born and growing up in the digital world, including what is happening in the brain and the sphere of emotional regulation. It is hard to disagree with the authors in this regard.

Questions about the impact of computerization of life and ubiquitous information and communication technology on the nature of man and his psychosocial development seem obvious, but at the same time difficult to resolve. Media discussions mainly revolve around the threat posed by spending many hours in front of a screen for the mental health of children and adolescents. The adult world seems to see potential danger where young people see their reality. Granic et al. (2020) note that children and adolescents who are maturing in the digital age have adapted so quickly to messengers such as WhatsApp, Instagram, Facebook, WeChat, Snapchat, TikTok, Twitter, Medium, YouTube, etc. that political, legal, psychological, sociological or scientific discourses are not keeping up with it. European statistics show that over 90% of children and adolescents from different European countries use the Internet every day (Eurostat, 2021). Young people use online and digital resources several times more often than adults to maintain contact, learn, seek opinions, buy, entertain and acquire knowledge – thus activities influencing the determination of their own interests, preferences or social attitudes. This is reflected in the educational offers that appear on the market. In schools, you can educate yourself in esports, game programming, as well as shaping the skills of creating your own image on the web, building visual identity and acquiring valuable fans (vlogger classes). The developing self finds its kind of continuity in the digital space. What is physically tangible more and more often begins to smoothly merge with what is virtual and tangible online, creating one whole. A whole that seems to be more than the sum of these elements.

Hybrid development

The presence of modern technologies in everyday life changes the educational, upbringing and, above all, development perspective. Suresh and Glenda (2018) point out that the availability and usefulness of the Internet mean that the ability to search and remember where to find on the Internet becomes a more important development competence than the ability to use the knowledge obtained from this source. The Internet is starting to be a tool that stimulates the development of cognitive functions in a specific direction. Creativity, multitasking, placing most of the necessary information in the online space is a kind of external memory of modern generations. In their meta-analysis, Suresh and Glenda (2018) also point out that online science itself has transformed. The content is more personalized and meets the user's needs. By giving the opportunity to interact, they engage children and adolescents. This commitment fosters the development of the ability to use social media, the Internet or digital messaging as forms of modern thinking, remembering and information processing. In this situation, the obvious consequence seems to be the introduction of modern technologies in upbringing and education. The effectiveness of these forms, however, depends on how much modern technologies serve to achieve clearly defined goals for students, and the teachers themselves are able to use this type of technology (Sivalingam and Subbaiyan, 2018; Suresh and Glenda, 2018).

Granic et al., (2020) propose that the development of modern children and adolescents should be considered in a model they describe as hybrid. Undoubtedly, it is difficult to disagree with researchers that nowadays the separation of the internal from the external becomes a challenge. The authors' model assumes that young people grow in an ecosystem of mutually interpenetrating physical and digital worlds. This applies to the intrapsychic space, in which an important element of identity development is the power of agency and the sense of coherence, as well as the effective fulfillment of social needs (especially belonging and acceptance). This idea also applies to the world of interpersonal relations, in which Granic et al., (2020) indicate the special importance of experiences related to being actively listened to, the possibility of developing stories about oneself and the world through elaboration, or awareness of inaccuracies (grappling contradictions). After all, online and offline are currently reflected in attempts to integrate man and his environment, providing a range of alternative narratives about oneself and the world (Granic et al., 2020).

Courage and the ability to achieve your own goals are competencies that are not easy to develop, especially in the period of adolescence, when it is natural to feel uncertainty and numerous doubts. In everyday life, it's not easy to be an action movie superhero. As research from recent years shows, however, playing video games may help in building agency competence through the possibility of multiple attempts, regardless of the final effect. Granic et al., (2020) emphasize that the success experienced by a young person in online games, rewarded effort and repeated attempts may moderate a positive attitude and, consequently, affect better educational achievements and well-being. The authors' analyses of various games available on the market are particularly interesting. The ability to identify with heroes experiencing difficult emotions, struggling with their shadow and almost unattainable goal and their story undoubtedly – as suggested by Granic et al., (2020) – shapes the private story of young people about themselves. However, one may wonder whether the specific blurring of the boundary between online and offline does not favor a certain continuity of this experience in both worlds: real and digital. However, it seems that transferring experiences from one world to another is mutual. In addition to drawing strength from the history of the Internet or gaming idol, it is also easy to become excessively convinced that the impossible is being realized. Perhaps this is one of the reasons for the almost immediate transfer of behaviors and emotions observed by children and adolescents in the world of the screen to offline reality. Every now and then there are media reports that children and adolescents imitate the behavior of the heroes of popular series or online games. The problem begins, however, when an adolescent experiencing his greatness on the Internet or social media is confronted with failure in the world of direct social relations. With a weakened and shaky ego, such a specific split may increase the risk of anxiety and depressive symptoms, and, as a consequence, mental decompensation. A protective factor in this respect, according to Granic et al., (2020) there may be a sense of coherence. A feeling that nowadays – according to the authors – is built in a continuous time based on the history of changes plotted and recorded in the media space (social media, blogs, etc.).

As the authors of the model also point out, social media can contribute to building and strengthening relationships, and thus social competencies. You are more anonymous on the web, you can feel safe, create a virtual self, a specific avatar. It is a space for creating and sharing narratives, especially motivating and attractive for stimulus-seekers. The world of internet games, video games and social media is extremely diverse. Depending on the nature of the interactive form of digital exchange, it can be both a space where you can train such skills as competition or competition, as well as a field for development and experiencing a sense of community, mutual care and cooperation (Granic et al., 2020). As Globokar (2018) points out, online forms of contact can be a valuable resource in a situation where people are separated by distance and constitute an additional form of contact, facilitating the maintenance of an already established relationship.

On the other hand, it is much more difficult to resolve conflicts or resolve misunderstandings online. It is easier to get negative comments or experience violence and harassment from others. The feeling of being ignored or excluded on the Internet, called cyber-ostracism, may contribute to a deterioration of mood, a decrease in self-esteem, belonging, social acceptance and finally self-importance (Bryant, 2018; Schneider et al., 2017). The analyses collected by Ersoy (2019) suggest that the most common – in terms of a negative effect – contemporary generations of children encounter online are:

- Cyberbullying or online harassment (suffering from disclosing private data, disseminating false information, humiliating and insulting others, sexting),
- Facebook depression (related to spending too much time on social networking websites and loosening relationships with loved ones or the fear of losing internet relationships and likes),
- Defective social relationship (resulting from dependence on social media, and thus stress in the face of face to face contact; difficulties in differentiating social relations).

As indicated by Nesi et al., (2020), the entry of ITC in human life also changed the nature of the sought-after social acceptance. Currently, a young person shapes his social status on the basis of the number of likes or positive comments left under his entries on the web and posted photos or artifacts. In a way, it can be said that it is not what you achieve, but how you present yourself in the media that matters. The hybrid world is a world in which development needs are alternately realized online and offline. The same applies to the individual elements of shaping identity, including rebellion, and also searching for oneself. Nesi et al., (2020) point out that, however, to create a coherent narrative about oneself, it is necessary to consciously integrate oneself into a whole. The authors discuss the growing share of digital spaces in the process of developing their own identity. However, they indicate that digital spaces are based on a finite algorithm. The behavior of users is in some way prompted and guided by this algorithm. The strength of a developed, own narrative lies in the conscious choice and decision of what should be remembered and integrated, and what should be forgotten. This would mean that, in this sense, digital technology and being online cannot replace direct experience and some part of yourself related to what is known as the conscious Self.

The model of Granic et al., (2020) also draws attention to the hybrid dimension of interpersonal and cultural space. Values, stories and messages are no longer found in fairy tales, but during listening to podcasts or online workshops. It is also worth remembering that online is a world where borders do not exist. With one click you can be on the other side of the world and watch other people's lives live. With the feeling of being part of a larger whole, it is easy to use digital technology to have access to alternative narratives, human choices and even an alternative world (Nesi et al., 2020).

Pandemic experience and human development

During the COVID-19 pandemic, humans have acquired a specific dimension in the context of offline-online reality. The generation of people undergoing a pandemic, not only born in isolation resulting from the coronavirus but also growing up in family and life crises, aggravated in the pandemic, came to be referred to as Generation Crown, Quaranteens or Illenials. The very attempts to separate the COVID-19 generation raise controversy (Rudolph and Zacher, 2020). Nevertheless, attention is drawn to the need to look at the specifics of human functioning in isolation from direct physical contact and the increased online functioning that is observed during a pandemic.

A systematic review conducted by Nearchou et al., (2020) indicated that the pandemic affects the mental health of children and adolescents, which is mainly visible in the intensification of anxiety symptoms, depressed mood, and problems with motivation. Stress, worry and fear of infection are factors that predispose to the emergence or worsening of psychopathological symptoms and behaviour problems. The authors of the systematic review point out that the isolation caused by the coronavirus will mainly affect the group of children and adolescents between the ages of 5 and 18. In the case of younger children, the stress experienced by their relatives will be more important. In the case of young people, the authors point out the danger of more frequent use of social media by this group. The authors suggest that more frequent exposure to social media in this age group, and thus to all kinds of information related to the pandemic, may increase – as in adults – the risk of developing depressive and/ or anxiety symptoms.

Adolescence is a time where physical and hormonal changes overlap with emotional and psychosocial changes. These changes, including the weakening and strengthening of individual nerve connections, occur in response to social experiences, environmental and cultural factors. Brazilian researchers compare the experiences of a pandemic to a crisis or even trauma. In their opinion, the long-term effects of stress caused by the pandemic may be mainly caused by children and adolescents living in crowded apartments, struggling with their own deficits and problems in their family life. Isolation, the inability to play, changing the environment, and the lack of support are additional risk factors that cannot be ignored, especially in childhood and adolescence. According to de Figuieredo et al., (2021), even a short-term exposure to stress, helplessness, neglect, violence, sensory deprivation and dysregulation of habits may result in disturbances in the functioning of the hypothalamic-pituitary-adrenal axis. By adopting the researchers' model, it can be assumed that children and adolescents developing in a pandemic will mature in a critical period of development in a different biological context. The open question is to what extent they will adapt to this change and to what extent it will have its long-term consequences. The model of Brazilian researchers assumes that these long-term effects will occur and that children growing up in a pandemic will be more likely to present psychopathological symptoms.

It is worth noting, however, that humans, especially children and adults, have the ability to adapt. The ability to regulate one's emotions during a pandemic (emotional regulation) obviously depends on the immediate environment, including the style of upbringing or support of loved ones (Domínguez-Álvarez et al., 2020). It would seem that a crisis such as a pandemic, especially a lockdown or quarantine, limiting the stay mainly to online and increasing the risk of disorders. However, children also have the capacity to self-regulate. They influence the environment and show the ability to experiment in everyday life. This ability, observed by clinicians, is not always appreciated by scientists. This potential is indicated, inter alia, by the analyses conducted by Bahia et al. (2020). The researchers were surprised to find that the Lability/Negativity ratios were less pronounced in children in quarantine than in those tested before quarantine. Thus, they found that, despite the precarious and unclear situation, children are capable of using resources (such as the availability of parents) or searching for new ones. Thus, they are able to survive even the most unpredictable and crisis situations.

It is worth noting at this point that the research on which the authors looked, like this book, were written at a time when the pandemic was ongoing. It is difficult to disagree with the assumption of Rudolph and Zacher (2020) that any predictions about whether this specific time has changed people enough to make it possible to speak of their different specificity is a speculation. Undoubtedly, however, the time of isolation or quarantine, which is slowly becoming a permanent element of the pandemic, in the case of young people, means more time spent in front of the screen. Thus, modern technologies mediate even more strongly in satisfying the natural need of belonging and contact with others, as well as building self-presentation during adolescence. However, this type of activity is also associated with the intense reaction of the anterior cingulate cortex (ACC), which is responsible, among others, for information processing and enforcement. Thus, each feedback in the online world causes a specific disturbance in the brain plane (cf. Crone and Konijn, 2018). It seems that with frequent and repetitive sequences of this kind, this kind of interaction becomes a kind of developmental pattern. Young people, therefore, do not develop simultaneously in the world of direct physical contacts and virtual reality. Nowadays, they take into account the context of the times in which we live, these two worlds are interconnected, and human development takes place in a combined manner in the interpenetrating offline and online spaces. The pandemic and its psychosocial consequences have exacerbated this trend.

Digital touch

The reality in which man functions more and more often today raises the question of whether the future of man is associated with a complete transition to the virtual sphere. After all, man is essentially a social being. While it is quite easy to imagine communication with others via social media or other modern technological achievements today, it is much more difficult to decide whether a person is able to function without physical contact with others.

Previous studies on the relationship between newborns and their caregivers have strengthened the belief that physical contact is the basis for growth, shaping responsiveness skills, empathy, finally a safe base and a safe attachment style (Bowlby, 1958; Bigelow and Williams, 2020; Norholt, 2020). Touch is the first communication tool that allows you to develop your potential and express the emotions you experience. Through the skin, a person experiences the world around him, especially in early childhood. Physical contact with oneself and the environment is an essential skill in fetal life and in the following years of life. Bigelow and Williams (2020) note that through physical contact, infants and their caregivers learn about each other and develop awareness about themselves and each other.

Skin-to-skin contact, as well as all forms of wearing, hugging and physical experiences constitute the basis of social touch – contact serving to build and maintain social bonds. Social touch is a whole, complex system of psycho-physiological reactions. It is based on the action of specialized sensory receptors and unmyelinated peripheral afferent fibers (C-touch, or CT fibers), which react preferentially to a gentle touch, stroking or temperature close to the temperature of the human body. It is assumed to trigger a number of physiological reactions (such as the secretion of oxytocin, serotonin) and psychological ones (feeling of pleasure, community and relaxation) (Cascio et al., 2019; Saarinen et al., 2021). These processes and the corresponding pathways in the nervous system mediate the formation of simple and more complex social bonds. All these systems are embedded in a specific and specific context – environment, social setting and culture (Cascio et al., 2019). In a broader perspective, social touch is not only a specific way of touching. In a broader sense, it is any intentional physical contact with another person with an emotional color (Saarinen et al., 2021). Therefore, it can be both a love hug and a high-five or a thrust with your hand.

The way people come into physical contact with each other and who they admit to each other also varies depending on the stage of development. The image of a newborn clinging to the mother's breast, or of being cuddled most of the time by an adult infant, gives way to more pragmatic physical contact in toddlers-adults relationships. As time goes on, social touch begins to be more and more aware and played in relationships with specific people. In the pre-school and school period, the experience of nursing touch and physical contact through play, especially in relation to the family, develops. As pointed out by

Cascio et al., (2019) friendly, gratifying physical closeness on the part of parents as well as other authorities (such as teachers) during this period is an important factor supporting development and increasing operational efficiency. In turn, in the period of adolescence and adulthood, intimate physical contact becomes more important, and the touch in interpersonal relationships begins to be consciously controlled. The repertoire of emotions that accompany social touch increases. Saarinen et al., (2021) point out that these are not necessarily positive feelings. In physical contact with another person, you can not only experience pleasure, love, support, but also jealousy, anger, crossing borders. With increasing self-awareness, it can paradoxically become more and more difficult to find someone to whom social touch is directed, and who has similar preferences. Whether social touch will be a pleasant and supportive experience for both sides of the contact depends – as Saarinen et al., (2021) point out – on the modulating influence of psychosocial factors such as toucher's characteristics (quality of relationship with the person who is touched, facial expressions, prejudices and group) membership of toucher, physical attractiveness) and factors related to the situational context (attentiveness to touch exposure, multimodal environment, person's exposure to distress or sensory pain).

The issue grew even more complex during the pandemic where, for health reasons, limiting physical contact with people became a recommendation, and sometimes the only possible choice. In this period, social contact was reduced even more to communication using ICT (messengers, applications, electronic devices). However, is this kind of communication able to replace the physical aspect of social touch? Are people able to grow and develop without being physically touched?

Previous studies have shown that the deprivation of physical touch can lead to aggressive behavior, school difficulties, developmental regression in children, and in adults to symptoms of anxiety, depression and worse well-being (von Mohr et al., 2021). von Mohr et al. (2021), analyzing the data obtained from over 1700 respondents, concluded that intimate contact (as one of the components of social touch, next to friendly touch and professional touch) may be a protective factor during the isolation that resulted from the pandemic. The authors of the research noticed that the desire for intimacy (hugs, kisses, caresses) is stronger the longer the period of isolation. This mainly affects people with anxious attachment. In contrast, those with avoidant attachment showed less need for tactile support and a tactile experience during physical isolation. These studies looked at pandemic isolation, but in fact do not appear to be unique to COVID-19 times. It seems that the reality in which communication is necessarily shifting more and more into the online sphere, paradoxically the lack of physical contact will not be such a big problem for people with insecure attachment style. This is confirmed, for example, by reports that people with insecure attachment style find in online contact a way to establish or maintain interpersonal relationships in a way that does not threaten their own self (Nitzburg and Farber, 2013; Trub, 2016).

The answer to the question whether it is possible to switch to online contact completely is still pending at the time of writing this book. An open question is to what extent "virtual contact" will be sufficient and to what extent man will adapt to it in evolution. de Figueiredo et al. (2021) point out that the brain is highly plastic, especially during childhood and adolescence. However, they emphasize that this plasticity also means susceptibility to stressors and mental health difficulties and that environmental and cultural factors have a moderating influence in this regard.

The demand for tactile contact in the virtual contact space is also being met by the data transmission, collection and processing systems that we use on a daily basis (ICT). After the period of adapting devices to the possibility of using the sense of touch in the reception of information (the so-called discriminative touch), for example through vibrating telephones or specific shapes of devices through which we communicate, the time has come to introduce affective and social touch to ICT. van Erp and Toet (2015) point out that most intelligent applications used by humans to support the social context of communication are based on visual and auditory information. At the same time, they point out that even simple interfaces, robots or other products of technology, including the possibility of kinesthetic and tactile experiences, can provide a mediated social touch, evoking a physiological, emotional and intellectual response in people participating in this type of contact. As a result, numerous devices are beginning to be produced with the aim of providing a person with sensations imitating contact with human skin of various structures, the human body at a certain temperature, and finally also with various forms of movement and types of touch (Jewitt et al., 2021b; Prattichizzo, 2021). Some researchers point to the value of this type of technology in securing the need for social touch in a situation of physical distance, such as isolation resulting from a disease or a pandemic (Jewitt et al., 2021). It is debatable, however, to what extent they are able to replace the developmental stimulation provided by direct contact with another human being.

Imagining devices and entire complex systems that mediate various forms of touch (such as stroking, massage, pressure, tickling, hand-to-hand contact, hand-holding, intimate touch) is real at the time of writing this book. Such ideas are now not only implemented in various areas of everyday life but also in science (van Erp and Toet, 2015; Jewitt et al., 2021). In the treatment process, intelligent robots are used both in medical procedures and in the educational process. Telepresence robots (combining physical and remote presence) are promoted as an excellent solution for the process of remote education, maintaining social contact in places where there are patients who are difficult to visit, or showing around potential places of stay (e.g., hospitals) (van Erp and Toet, 2015). Medical simulation centers that allow the reconstruction of treatment rooms, along with robots imitating patients and members of the medical service, will probably be a standard in teaching medical professions in a few years' time. Reproducing medical procedures and operations creates the possibility of shaping technical skills, but also communication competencies necessary for future work with the patient. The ability to record the practiced forms of reaction and debriefing shapes the awareness of oneself as a future representative of the aid professions. It also seems to be an excellent solution in an ethical context. Future medics will eventually practice under safe and controlled conditions, prior to contact with the patient in reality. It is a Solomonic solution, taking into account the challenge of clinical intervention of a young adept of medical art and the stress of the person in the role of the patient.

More puzzling are reports of new applications, prototypes of remote communication, interfaces for maintaining close, intimate relationships between people using the sense of touch. Various portable devices are quite commonly used that allow you to send messages about support, emotions and longing to others through an appropriate touch/pressure of the screen. It is enough for the partner of the interaction to compress or properly touch, for example, a necklace, bracelet or watch (Hey Touch type) for the other side of this relationship to feel the touch through their device (Ley and Rambukkana, 2021). An example is teledildonics devices. They allow you to experience sexual intimacy with your partner without their physical presence through remote operation or online synchronization. Kissenger is also arousing more and more research interest – a mobile application with an attachment that allows kissing, analyzing the physical aspects of a kiss and receiving it using a similar attachment by the recipient of the kiss. Following the manufacturer's information, it can be assumed that this device was intended to support close contact between people who are at a physical distance. Over time, however, Kissenger prototypes appeared, enabling haptic kissing sensations through the Internet to be in contact with robots or avatars (Cheok and Zhang, 2019). The authors of the prototype assume that the emotional and intimate relationships between humans and robots, based on e.g. on artificial intelligence, it is basically a matter of the near future. Transferring what has so far been available only in physical form to the real world, in their opinion, will initiate the development of new behaviors, concepts, culture and relationships in a previously unimaginable way. Therefore, they suggest that the development of artificial intelligence should go towards the development of emotional intelligence, with optimism assuming that ultimately humans and robots will communicate on an emotional level, establish intimate relationships, and bestow love and empathy (Cheok and Zhang, 2019).

This is where the question arises about the purpose and direction of this type of activity. Is the need for closeness, and at the same time for shaping relationships in a safe, satisfying, almost ideal way so strong in the modern man? Or vice versa, it is a response to the hunger for physical experiences, the presence of others in the process of inevitable transformation that man is undergoing today, not only technologically, biologically, but also psychologically. Undoubtedly, the perception of physical presence increases the sense of community, one's social identity and fulfills social needs. This is indicated by the reflections of the participants of the workshops devoted to the creation of new technologies, registered by Jewitt et al., (2021b). A review of the discussions recorded by the authors gives rise to a reflection that the creation of reality is dominated not only by the desire for the tangibility of physical contact, its availability, but also the possibility of reaching for contact that is in readiness, which can be controlled and disciplined in some way. Partly based on this belief, activities aimed at introducing touch in virtual space are also carried out indirectly. There are devices that allow us to meet and physically contact in virtual space through avatars. With the use of simple devices (artificial hand), people are able to meet in virtual reality (e.g. a game) in a certain illusion of bodily contact. They can interact with each other through their avatars or agents. Introducing this aspect of contact into a virtual relationship contributes to experiences close to people and blurs the boundaries between a human and a computer (Hoppe et al., 2020). Research also indicates that digital touch as mediated social touch can modulate sympathy, the sense of sharing a common experience, and regulate physiological responses. First of all, however, due to the proven therapeutic utility of the relationship between people and social robots or social agents in the form of virtual agents on screen, research is being carried out on the value of introducing tactile modality into this type of relationship. The idea is to shape the capacity for empathic communication in robots, avatars and agents involved in relationships with people.

Towards the borders

All the described changes open up a number of questions about the limits of functioning in virtual reality, mediated by social touch and the ethics of these developmental changes. Who is responsible for mediated contact by ICT products? How to translate such a complex and difficult to grasp context of consent to contact into this type of relationship? To what extent is this room for abuse? How to protect personal boundaries and yourself in a reality where boundaries cease to exist? After all, what is developmental and what is dysfunctional in this new context? These are questions that should be driven by further socio-political research and activities (Jewitt et al., 2021a; Ley and Rambukkana, 2021). Taking a closer look at this issue, participants of the digital social touch design workshops, described by Jewitt et al., (2021a), developed the Manifesto for Digital Social Touch in Crisis (Jewitt et al., 2021a). Its purpose was to determine a specific map, key points for designers, programmers and researchers focusing on introducing human functioning into the online reality. They pointed out the need to be guided by the following principles in further research, research and implementation of touch into modern technologies:

- Make Social Touch Centre,
- Design Touch First, Technology Second,
- Democratize Touch: Don't Lock It In,
- Keep Touch Private and Secure by Design,
- Move Beyond Vibration: Feel Beyond the Habituated,
- Foster Exploration of Meaningful Touch Experiences,
- Remake, Don't Only Replicate!,
- Manage Great "Tech-Xpectations",
- Develop Open Touchy Tools,
- Keep Speculating.

The authors of the Manifesto pointed out that all attempts to include tactile modality in virtual experiences should be interdisciplinary, creative, open to experimentation, based on a common conceptual system and shared resources, tools, and should respect human privacy and intimacy, and be diverse, take into account the cultural context, interaction, openness to modification and, above all, be discussed and regulated at the same time.

The transition of social touch to digital touch seems inevitable but leaves clinical questions for what and what consequences it will have for the psychological sphere of a human being. van Erp and Toet (2015) view these kinds of changes with optimism. They recognize that when the difficulties at the interface of modern ICT technologies and psychology are successfully resolved, digital touch can contribute to improving the quality of life, bridging the gap between the real and virtual world and making artificial entities similar to human existence. From a philosophical point of view, however, as indicated by Ley and Rambukkana (2021), the human body is both a subject and an object that realizes man through his physical relationship with the world. In their opinion, technologically mediated touch differs and will be different from direct physical contact in that it is limited by the technology's capabilities and de facto requires tuning to it (and not vice versa or mutually). However, they also point out that with time all devices imitating touch may become so precise that they almost imperceptibly become a natural extension of the body. They will, in a way, start to be treated as an element of reality and everyday life. By developing this idea, one can therefore predict that a man will in a way expand his boundaries, he will also develop not so much through the development of technology that is his work, but in it as part of himself. As a consequence, it will become hybrid to some extent. This developmental trajectory is happening right before our eyes. The line between what we used to define real and what is virtual is becoming more and more blurred. If this trend continues, it can be assumed that all human attributes and competencies, including the attachment to others' patterns, will also become hybrid to some extent. Even if this issue is still debatable, it will certainly have to be answered by considerations and research in the field of developmental psychology. It is difficult to imagine any development paradigm today without taking into account the key role of the digital part of human existence.

References

Bahia, A.F., Martins, C., Bitencourt, A. (2020). #stayathome?: Increased children's emotion regulation in covid-19 pandemic. *Estudos de Psicologia (Natal)*, 25(2), 232–242. DOI: 10.22491/1678-4669.20200023

Baltes, P.B. (1987). Theoretical Propositions of Life-Span Developmental Psychology: On the Dynamics Between Growth and Decline. *Developmental Psychology*, 23(5), 611–626. DOI: 10.1037/0012-1649.23.5.611

Bigelow, A.E., Williams, L.R. (2020). To have and to hold: Effects of physical contact on infants and their caregivers. *Infant Behavior & Development*, 61, 101494. DOI: 10.1016/j.infbeh.2020.101494

Bowlby J. (1958). The nature of the child's tie to the mother. *The International Journal of Psycho-Analysis*, 39(5), 350–373.

Brillet, F., Hulin, A., Leroy, J., Bourliataux-Lajoinie, S. (2011). E-generation, What's New? *Journal of Human Ressources Management Research*, 1–15. DOI: 10.5171/2011.784128

Bryant, A. (2018). *The Effect of Social Media on the Physical, Social Emotional, and Cognitive Development of Adolescents*. Honors Senior Capstone Projects. 37. https://scholarworks.merrimack.edu/honors_capstones/37

Buckingham, D. (2006). Is there a digital generation? In: D. Buckingham, R. Willet (eds.) *Digital Generations Children, Young People, and the New Media*. UK: Routledge.

Cascio, C.J., Moore, D., McGlone, F. (2019). Social touch and human development. *Developmental Cognitive Neuroscience*, 35, 5–11. DOI: 10.1016/j.dcn.2018.04.009

Cascio, C.J., Moore, D., McGlone, F. (2019). Social touch and human development. *Developmental Cognitive Neuroscience*, 35, 5–11. DOI: 10.1016/j.dcn.2018.04.009

Cheok, A.D., Zhang, E.Y. (2019). Kissenger: Transmitting Kiss Through the Internet. In: A. D. Choek, E. Y. Zhang (eds.), *Human–Robot Intimate Relationships* (pp. 77–97). London: Springer.

Crone, E.A., Konijn, E.A. (2018). Media use and brain development during adolescence. *Nature Communications*, 9(1), 588. DOI: 10.1038/s41467-018-03126-x

Domínguez-Álvarez, B., López-Romero, L., Gómez-Fraguela, J.A., Romero, E. (2020). Emotion regulation skills in children during the COVID-19 pandemic: Influences on specific parenting and child adjustment. *Revista de Psicología Clínica con Niños y Adolescentes*, 7(3), 81–87. DOI: 10.21134/rpcna.2020.mon.2042

Ersoy, M. (2019). Social Media and Children In: G. Sari, M. Ersoy, (eds.) *Handbook of Research Children's Consumption Technology IGI Global*, (pp. 11–24). USA. DOI: 10.4018/978-1-5225-5733-3.ch002

Eurostat, (2021). *Youth online: a way of life*. Pobrane z: https://ec.europa.eu/eurostat/statistics-explained/index.php?title=Being_young_in_Europe_today_-_digital_world#Youth_online:_a_way_of_life (11.02.2022)

de Figueiredo, C.S., Sandre, P.C., Portugal, L., Mázala-de-Oliveira, T., da Silva Chagas, L., Raony, Í., Ferreira, E.S., Giestal-de-Araujo, E., Dos Santos, A.A., & Bomfim, P.O. (2021). COVID-19 pandemic impact on children and adolescents' mental health: Biological, environmental, and social factors. *Progress in Neuro-psychopharmacology & Biological Psychiatry*, 106, 110171. DOI: 10.1016/j.pnpbp.2020.110171

Galapathy, P., Wathurapatha, W., Ranasinghe, P., Wijayabandara, M.D.M.S., Warapitiya, D.S., Weerasuriya, K. (2017). The (e-Generation): The Technological Usage and Experiences of Medical Students from a Developing Country. *International Journal of Telemedicine and Applications*, 1–6. DOI: 10.1155/2017/6928938

Globokar, R. (2018). Impact of digital media on emotional, social and moral development of children. *Nova Prisutnost*. XVI, 560-560. DOI: 10.31192/np.16.3.8

Granic, I., Morita, H., Scholten, H., (2020). Beyond Screen Time: Identity Development in the Digital Age. *Psychological Inquiry*, 31, 195–223. DOI: 10.1080/1047840X.2020.1820214

Green, M.G., Piel, J.A. (2016). *Theories of Human Development: A Comparative Approach.* NY: Routladge.

Hoppe, M., Rossmy, B., Neumann, D.P., Streuber, S., Schmidt, A., Machulla, T.K. (2020). A Human Touch: Social Touch Increases the Perceived Human-likeness of Agents in Virtual Reality. Conference on Human Factors in Computing Systems, 1–11. DOI: 10.1145/3313831.3376719

Jewitt, C., Price, S., Steimle, J., Huisman, G., Golmohammadi, L., Pourjafarian, N., Frier, W., Howard, T., Askari, S.I., Ornati, M., Panëels, S., Weda, J. (2021a). Manifesto for Digital Social Touch in Crisis. *Frontiers in Computer Science*, 3. DOI: 10.3389/fcomp.2021.754050

Jewitt, C., Leder, Mackley, K., Price, S. (2021b). Digital touch for remote personal communication: An emergent sociotechnical imaginary. *New Media & Society*, 23(1), 99–120. DOI: 10.1177/1461444819894304

Lerner, R.M., Lerner, J.V., Bowers, E.P., Geldhof, G.J. (2015a). Positive youth development and relational-developmental-systems. In: W. F. Overton, P. C. M. Molenaar, R. M. Lerner (eds.), *Handbook of Child Psychology and Developmental Science: Theory and Method* (pp. 607–651). New York: John Wiley & Sons, Inc.

Lerner, R.M., Hershberg, R.M., Hilliard, L.J., Johnson S.K. (2015b). Human Development, J. Wright (eds.) Theories of. In: *International encyclopedia of social and behavioral sciences* (pp. 276–282). Oxford: Elsevier. DOI: 10.1016/B978-0-08-097086-8.34017-X

Ley, M., Rambukkana, N. (2021). Touching at a Distance: Digital Intimacies, Haptic Platforms, and the Ethics of Consent. *Science and Engineering Ethics*, 27(5), 63. DOI: 10.1007/s11948-021-00338-1

Nearchou, F., Flinn, C., Niland, R., Subramaniam, S.S., Hennessy, E. (2020). Exploring the Impact of COVID-19 on Mental Health Outcomes in Children and Adolescents: A Systematic Review. *International Journal of Environmental Research and Public Health*, 17(22), 8479. DOI: 10.3390/ijerph17228479

Nesi, J., Telzer, E.H., Prinstein, M.J. (2020). Adolescent Development in the Digital Media Context. *Psychological Inquiry*, 31(3), 229–234. DOI: 10.1080/1047840x.2020.1820219

Nitzburg, G.C., Farber, B.A. (2013). Putting up emotional (Facebook) walls? Attachment status and emerging adults' experiences of social networking sites. *Journal of Clinical Psychology*, 69(11), 1183–1190. DOI: 10.1002/jclp.22045

Norholt, H. (2020). Revisiting the roots of attachment: A review of the biological and psychological effects of maternal skin-to-skin contact and carrying of full-term infants. *Infant Behavior & Development*, 60. DOI: 10.1016/j.infbeh.2020.101441

Prattichizzo, D. (2021). Beyond the Pandemic: The Role of Haptics in Defining the New Normal. *IEEE Transcriptions on Haptics*, 14(1), 1. DOI: 10.1109/TOH.2021.3065772

Rudolph, C.W., Zacher, H. (2020). *"The COVID-19 Generation": A Cautionary Note.* Work, Aging and Retirement, waaa009. DOI: 10.1093/workar/waaa009

Saarinen, A., Harjunen, V., Jasinskaja-Lahti, I., Jääskeläinen, I.P., Ravaja, N. (2021). Social touch experience in different contexts: A review. *Neuroscience & Biobehavioral Reviews*, 131, 360–372. DOI: 10.1016/j.neubiorev.2021.09.027

Schneider, F.M., Zwillich, B., Bindl, M.J., Hopp, F.R., Reich, S., Vorderer, P. (2017). Social media ostracism: *The effects of being excluded online. Computers In Human Behavior*, 385. DOI: 10.1016/j.chb.2017.03.052

Sivalingam, D., Subbaiyan, M. (2018). The modern technology are using education for adolescents. *Journal of Applied and Advanced Research*, 3(1), 1. DOI: 10.21839/jaar.2018.v3 iS1.155

Suresh C.J., Glenda, R. (2018). Information Technology, Internet Use, and Adolescent Cognitive Development. *International Conference on Computational Systems and Information Technology for Sustainable Solutions.* DOI: 10.1109/CSITSS.2018.8768780

Trub, L. (2016). A Portrait of the Self in the Digital Age: Attachment, Splitting, and Self-Concealment in Online and Offline Self-Presentation. *Psychoanalytic Psychology.* Advanceonline publication. DOI: 10.1037/pap0000123

van Erp, J.B.F., Toet, A. (2015). Social Touch in Human–Computer Interaction. *Frontiers in Digital Humanities*, 2, 1–14. DOI: 10.3389/fdigh.2015.00002.

von Mohr, M., Kirsch, L.P., Aikaterini, F. (2021). Social touch deprivation during COVID-19: effects on psychological wellbeing and craving interpersonal touch. *The Royal Society*, 8, 210287210287 DOI: 10.1098/rsos.210287.

Wilson, S., Olino, T.M. (2021). A developmental perspective on personality and psychopathology across the life span. *Journal of Personalized Medicine*, 89(5), 915–932. DOI: 10.1111/jopy.12623

Chapter 2

Contemporary forms of establishing attachment

Chapter overview

The chapter is devoted to the phenomenon of attachment, the understanding of this construct in the context of changes to which man is subject in the era of digitization. It juxtaposes the existing theoretical concepts of attachment with contemporary research on this construct, both in terms of secure and insecure attachment. It deals with the topic of cultural attachment as a starting point for a discussion on the change that attachment undergoes in offline–online human functioning. The last part of the chapter is an invitation to consider to what extent the assumption about transferring the pattern of attachment developed in the real world to the attachment structure presented in the virtual world is fully justified. Research on how attachment is formed in the virtual world is not only discussed in the context of the use of electronic media but also other Information and Communications Technology (ICT) achievements (such as contact with avatars). It introduces the concept of E-attachment, as a proposal of a symbolic approach to the complexity of the construct in question in relation to traditional descriptions of attachment, and at the same time emphasizing its new, more complex dimension, shaped in the dynamically changing offline–online reality. The proposed model of thinking invites you to pose specific questions about the nature of attachment in the contemporary world as directions of future research in this field.

Attachment in human life

Attachment is a phenomenon that arouses the interest of both scientists and clinical practitioners. The human tendency to develop strong emotional bonds became the main subject of John Bolwby's interest, to whom psychiatrists, psychologists and psychotherapists refer to the theory of attachment to the present day. Attachment theory was created primarily to explain the influence of early childhood experiences in the relationship of the developing little person with people in his immediate environment on his later development and emotional and social functioning (Ainsworth, 2021). The specific type of

DOI: 10.4324/9781003221043-3

attachment, which cannot be described only in terms of closeness, is, however, an observed and intuitively recognized experience in tribal cultures, as well as in the natural world surrounding man. It takes place on several levels.

In the mid-20th century, Harlow proved that the comfort of contact with the mother is crucial for the development of the primate infant (1958). Skin-to-skin contact is in fact the first space in which attachment and mutual, responsive contact take place. These observations formed the starting point for the attachment theory. It is worth recalling that in its original form, the attachment theory referred to the observations of relationships between babies and mothers made by Bowlby, Ainsworth and their associates (Ainsworth and Bowlby, 1991; Ainsworth, 2021). Research on attachment influenced the development of the concept itself, as well as the ways of understanding it. Attachment is something other than bonding. It seems that the essence of attachment was aptly captured by Benoit (2004), who wrote that it appears and develops not only when a child treats its guardian and relationship with him as a basis for exploration but also uses it when he wants to take refuge or feel comfortable. Research conducted since the mid-20th century indicates that attachment is a process that may also apply to relatives other than the parents, and even to objects other than people. As it turns out, in shaping attachment, not only the predisposition to contact the child and his loved ones may be important but also biological (including genetic) factors, the environment and finally the socio-economic and cultural context (Yap et al., 2019).

The observations made by Bowlby led him to believe that the child, exposed to repeatedly losing contact with a significant person who was the mother and whom he trusted, will eventually begin to show difficulties in interpersonal relations, efficient emotional functioning and finally psycho-pathological symptoms. Thus, Bolwby recognized the specific bond between the young child and mother as the basis for shaping a complex construct called attachment, which was the kind of competence necessary for satisfactory growth and development (Ainsworth and Bowlby, 1991). The attachment itself is based on a strong biological and emotional bond and the search for this closeness both in the presence and absence of a person for whom a pattern of attachment behavior, observable by the environment, has been formed. In a way, attachment and the emerging attachment style equip a person for a further life journey, in a certain way, independence, a sense of security or the ability to derive satisfaction from relationships with others.

Bowlby's attachment behaviors were included in a number of other behaviors that were essential for the maintenance of life. The experiences of comfort and security (or lack thereof) from early childhood relationships are internalized in the form of internal working models of attachment. These, in turn, become the basis for shaping subsequent relationships with others. Functioning in a specific attachment style, implemented by a pattern of specific behaviors, creates specific conditions for the development of selected features and properties of the nervous system. Bowlby clearly indicated that attachment is not given, but is formed (from the phase of orientation and signals directed without distinguishing people, through the phase of orientation and signals directed to selected people, to maintaining closeness with the selected person by means of signals and locomotion) (Bowlby, 2021). He believed that the first years of life, during infancy and toddlerhood, were of key importance in this regard. According to Bowlby, a child comes into the world equipped with a system of basic behaviors, serving the communication of basic needs. Mary Ainsworth emphasized that the property of these basic skills of a child is the ability to synchronize, to react responsively to the environment (Ainsworth, 2021; Ainsworth and Bowlby, 1991). This ability is the beginning of the entire adventure of attachment.

John Bolwby assumed that we can talk about the developed ability to attach in a child at the age of about 6 months. Attachment behaviors then begin to be varied but also responsive. Thanks to the attachment theory, the concept of developmental separation anxiety and fear of strangers has become a permanent fixture in the considerations on the natural behavior of children in education or family counseling. The authors and followers of the attachment theory pointed out that although children differ in the quality of their anxiety response to separation or the appearance of others, they present these features until the age of two, somewhat regardless of the culture or environment in which they are brought up (Ainsworth, 2021).

Research on attachment, based on observations in natural and laboratory conditions (the so-called strange situation procedure), led Mary Ainswort to distinguish three main patterns of behavior, describing the way the relationship between infant and mother played out (B- securely attached; A- anxiously attached-avoidant, C- anxiously attached-resistant/ambilevant). In further research practice, subsequent subtypes of three basic patterns began to be observed and distinguished, depending on the severity and quality of the child's behavior, observed in the strange situation procedure. Nevertheless, they all refer to the secure attachment and the two distinct types of insecure attachment. Another additional group, called insecure-disorganized/disoriented attachment pattern (type D), was proposed by Main (Main and Solomon, 1986). These four basic specific attachment patterns have become firmly established in clinical and therapeutic thinking.

It is worth recalling here that secure attachment is a kind of attachment related to mutual responsiveness, a sense of security and comfort. It is manifested by maintaining relationships by the child, empathy and mindfulness of the closest caregiver (usually the mother), as well as seeking active support for the relatives in an ambiguous, stressful or threatening situation. The bond with the guardian, based on a sense of security, becomes a source of exploration by the child of his environment and building trust towards others, according to his/her own needs. With time, the adolescent child, internalizing this model, actively engages in relations with the environment, even in the absence of his "exemplary", closest guardian. It favors the further, proper development of the child, shapes his/her social skills, positive self-esteem, empathy, resilience, creativity and the ability to cope with difficult situations.

The avoidant attachment type is characterized by avoiding contact with a significant person by the child. Parallel to this avoidance, there is a reaction of lack of responsiveness, specific rejection or reluctance in the situation of a child seeking contact (Ainsworth, 2021; Benoit, 2004). As a consequence, it can be assumed that the developing child develops the belief that signaling himself can result in rejection and distance. This favors further avoidance. The child does not seek or stop looking for solace in the parent's arms. As a consequence, a person develops a distrustful attitude towards interpersonal relationships, as they do not give a sense of security and cannot be counted on.

The ambilevant attachment type is also characterized by distrust towards the environment and a slight willingness to explore it. In this case, the inconsistency and unpredictability of the caregiver's reactions go hand in hand with the child's tendency to react with anxiety to attempts at separation and, at the same time, to refuse to cradle it when it is undertaken. Extreme emotions and extreme, often exorbitant reactions are behaviors that can be observed in both a young child and an adolescent teenager. There is a conviction that only in this way one can be the center of attention and, consequently, gain a safe dependency for which there is a struggle, and also for which a constant anxiety is manifested.

All of the above types of attachments are organized in some way. However, there is a group of children that grows into a disorganized type of attachment. Their reactions seem to have an undiscovered intention or purpose. This type is sometimes referred to as "fright without solution". Atypical, contradictory, dissociated, confused, sometimes freeze-like behavior of a child is usually accompanied by unusual, dissociated, often frightening behavior of the closest caregiver. Such reactions are usually caused by untreated traumas and traumatic experiences, often accumulating during life and increasing the experienced stress (Duschinsky, 2018; Benoit, 2004).

It is worth noting that the founders of the theory of attachment were convinced of the durability of attachment patterns. However, they focused on observing children's behavior in relation to their caregivers. Research conducted among adults has brought knowledge about attachment styles in interpersonal relationships, mainly partnerships. Characteristics for these observations are taking into account not data from the observations, but above all the perspective of the examined person, both on the models and attachment behavior of one's own and other people. Such a combined approach was proposed by Bartholomew and Horowitz (Bartholomew and Shaver, 1998). Their two-dimensional model of positivity of self and other allowed for the emergence of four attachment styles: secure (low attachment anxiety, low attachment avoidance), preoccupied (high attachment anxiety, low attachment avoidance), dismissing (low attachment anxiety, high attachment avoidance), fearful (high attachment anxiety, high attachment avoidance) (Morales-Vives et al., 2021; Bartholomew and Shaver, 1998). Thus, adults with secure attachment present internalized self-worth and feel comfortable in close relationships. People with preoccupied attachment do not value themselves, but at times even desperately seek the acceptance of others, not feeling completely confident in these relationships. Dismissing attachment is often associated with avoiding others who are not viewed as a source of support. Leaning on oneself and on others, in turn, is not the property of those who are characterized by fearful attachment. With this type of attachment style, it's hard to talk about self-love, self-worth and trusting others.

The classification created by Bartholomew and Horowitz extended the possibilities of testing attachment with questionnaire methods proposed to adults. The ideas of Shaver and his colleagues, developed in the second half of the 20th century and continued in the 20th century, undoubtedly contributed to this (Mikulincer and Shaver, 2016; Mikulincer et al., 2003). Their essence is the assumption that the attachment developed from childhood through adulthood should be considered in the context of two dimensions: avoidance and anxiety. Avoidance refers to the degree of aversion towards others, discomfort in close and intimate relationships with others, and thus the possibility/inability to obtain support from others. A high avoidance index is associated with a tendency to use a strategy of denial of emotions, inhibiting emotional reactions perceived as a potential source of rejection. The dimension attachment anxiety refers to the severity of the fear of rejection, negative self-view. Consequently, it is associated with a tendency to use hyperactiviting strategies for emotional regulation, including exaggerated demands for care and contact with others (Mikulincer and Shaver, 2016). It is worth noting that although in general Shaver and colleagues and followers of their ideas use these two concepts – dimensions, in their works there were suggestions of typology resulting from the combination of the severity of avoidance and anxiety. The same happens in the case of adaptation or construction of subsequent questionnaires to study attachment by other authors (Mikulincer and Shaver, 2016; Pilkonis et al., 2013; Morales-Vives et al., 2021). This requires both the readers and the authors of various attachment works to be highly attentive to the context and understanding in which the terms avoidance, anxious or fearful are used. There is also a noticeable discrepancy between the reports based on the observations of children and parents and the observations derived from the declarations of adults. The disorganized attachment type is rarely mentioned when discussing the romantic styles of attachment in adulthood. With the diversity and complexity of the functioning of modern man, moving smoothly between online and offline, the complexity of the styles of attachment he presents also seems to be a natural consequence. This was already noted in the early 20st century by Stein et al., (2002). Their research indicated that most people display an attachment style that does not fit into the well-known and distinguished three/four categories. Moreover, it seems that in declarations (collected by questionnaires) adults tend to perceive themselves multidimensionally, as manifesting features of different attachment styles (Morales-Vives et al., 2021; Stein et al., 2002). Therefore, one wonders whether in this situation it would not be clearer to simply talk only about secure and insecure attachment styles.

The popularity of the theory of attachment has contributed to increased awareness of what is happening in the relationship between a small child and its caregivers, especially in the area of contact between the mother and the newborn child. The image of a responsive parent hugging a baby in a sling has become established in the common consciousness. Bowlby emphasized, however, that the warm and lasting relationship of intimacy between the child and the parent should be satisfactory for both of them (Bretherton, 1992).

It is worth noting that difficulties with attachment and the consequences of this fact in the future may result not only from low responsiveness or un-availability of significant people. In order to fulfill its function effectively, the attachment system must also be based on the child's innate or shaped ability to signal its needs or respond to the signals of the environment. A review of research conducted among children with intellectual disability indicates that they more often present insecure, often disorganized attachment styles (Vanwalleghem et al., 2021; Granqvist et al., 2017). Difficulty in expressing one's own emotions in adults, less emotional reactivity and less expressive facial expressions are elements that may make it difficult to grasp the emotional needs of children and provide sensitive responses to them. It is also possible to imagine a situation in which some children (e.g. diagnosed with genetic diseases) are naturally more prone to undifferentiated approach or impulsiveness or distance, which makes it difficult to form a safe base. Inherently, it is difficult to talk about the possibility of observing behaviors corresponding to a secure attachment style. Rather, they seem to reflect a specific style of functioning in a given disease. Undoubtedly, it is clear that neurocognitive deficits or dysfunctions are a risk factor for the development of insecure, mainly disorganized forms of attachment, and vice versa (Vanwalleghem et al., 2021; Pritchard et al., 2015). The open question, however, is still not whether this is the case, but how to distinguish one issue from another. Perhaps, as people with some kind of difficulty develop their attachment style based on other kinds of internal operating models? For example, those that seem completely functional in their context, although out of context, already make a different impression in the environment. A specific social, environmental and finally cultural context is something that applies to every adolescent child. Maturing in the age of technology, man differs not only in terms of needs but also in the ways of signaling his needs for closeness or a sense of security. Undoubtedly, he is someone for whom the use of modern technologies for the purposes of establishing relationships, entertainment, education or gaining support and help is something obvious (the so-called digital native) (Prensky, 2001; Parsons, 2017). Does this change also apply to the attachment structure itself? By changing, evolving, living in an extension of offline-online, does the secure attachment of modern man take the same form as in the times of J. Bolwby? These are the questions that still don't have a clear answer.

Cultural context of attachment

Clinicians from different countries used to think that secure attachment is the most common. Indeed, the mere observation of the fact of human development, overcoming successive crises by him or responding to successive environmental challenges could suggest that most human beings develop effective adaptation strategies that are assumed to be achieved through the experience of a secure attachment relationship. This seems to be confirmed by the analyzes of Mesman et al., (2016). They indicated that nearly 50–70% of the world's children (except in countries affected by extreme crises) show signs of secure attachment. The secure attachment force was also proven by the analyzes of Eder and colleagues (2021) conducted during the crisis and restrictions related to COVID-19 in Spain, Austria, Poland and the Czech Republic. Attachment security turned out to be the most important predictor of satisfaction in intimate relationships during the lockdown, to some extent independent of the stress resulting from pandemic restrictions.

A manifestation of secure attachment is not only openness to what is new but also the ability to refer to an internally internalized safe harbor when necessary. According to Strand et al., (2019), these two trends (novelty-seeking and security-seeking) also take place at the social level, thus not only differentiating societies but also their individual members. Collectivist societies appear to favor the disclosure and support of social-security-seeking behavior, thereby exposing anxious patterns. Individualist society, on the other hand, seems to strengthen messages, and thus social-novelty-seeking patterns, in which self-reliance is predominant and, in the extreme, the idea of not supporting the idea of trust in others (avoidant tendency) is dominant. Researchers emphasize that Western culture strengthens the attitudes and behaviors related to loneliness, lack of expression of emotions or seeking support in the process of education. They are perceived as evidence of the independence of the adolescent child. An additional factor enhancing the formation of insecure attachment patterns in the community, in parents, and consequently in children, is the repressive experience of socialization. Strand et al., (2019), pointing to this phenomenon, referred mainly to the experiences of national minorities. Researchers developed a two-way model of the relationship between culture and attachment. Cultural types are defined in some way by the types of attachment that dominate a given society. Attachment patterns, their character marked by culture are realized in families and thus passed on to the next generation. In this way, the transmitted patterns begin to be stable, similar in subsequent generations.

Culturally well-adapted people are therefore those who formed a base for both security-seeking and novelty-seeking in their early childhood. It is hard to disagree with the authors of this model who suggest that guardians' avoidance strategies invite children to ignore signals of seeking safety in children, thereby enhancing their avoidant strategies. However, the question arises whether we, as humans, are doomed to this determinism. It seems that especially in the face of a crisis such as a pandemic, it is easy to strengthen anxiety or avoidance attitudes. Their escalation may be the greater the lack of a safe base in life experience and in the child and the caregiver. On the other hand, in the next stages of life, we have the opportunity to create relationships that will strengthen a certain kind of our flexibility. As Rothbaum et al., (2000) emphasized at the beginning of the 21st century, it would be a mistake to juxtapose some cultural forms with others, and consequently some types of attachment to others. Therefore, it is difficult to talk about one universal theory of attachment. The differentiation in the views on what attachment is indicated in this chapter may de facto reflect the fact that people shape closer relationships and strengthen attachment patterns that allow them to adapt to different situations and contexts in which they live (Rothbaum et al., 2000).

As indicated in the meta-analysis by Opie et al., (2021) the most stable organization of attachment, also intergenerational, is security. Insecure attachment is less stable during development. Therefore, it seems that there is always a chance to gain corrective and base-strengthening experiences. Strand et al., (2019) proposed that attachment styles should be considered in the context of their strengths and weaknesses in relation to a given culture. This approach is conducive to the belief in the dynamics of attachment and to treating any attachment style as a potential resource in a given time and space of life. Granqvist (2021) emphasizes that the stability of secure attachment is a response to the needs of evolution. According to the researcher, it increases openness to socialization, plasticity, that is critical factors for cultural progress. Interesting is the understanding of attachment as a specific trigger of social learning, proposed by Granqvist (2021). His question about how important the mentalization processes are in the process of mutual relations between cultural transmission and attachment can be understood as a question about the primordial nature of attachment. Sensitivity and the ability to mentalize are undoubtedly important to a mutual relationship. Is it sufficient or necessary to shape a secure base? This is an open question. Assuming that attachment is a dynamic structure, it is natural to assume that its nature will change in the course of human evolution.

Neither the man nor the culture in which he functions is static. There is a specific bond between these two structures, referred to as "cultural attachment" (Yap et al., 2019). Yap et al., (2019) use this phenomenon to explain seemingly surprising human behavior, such as traveling hundreds of kilometers to eat food reminiscent of childhood times or reluctance to get rid of items that can be replaced with more functional or useful. According to the researchers, culture as a network of generational and also shared values, beliefs and meanings can be the basis for a secure attachment. The attachment shaped in the relationship with parents and caregivers can therefore be supplemented, buffered and possibly modified by cultural attachment (Yap et al., 2019; Hong et al., 2013). Culture gives people the opportunity to form groups, support, exchange experiences, and ensure individual and group survival. In culture, not only are roles given but also narratives about a sense of security and danger are created. These qualities of culture are indicated as providing grounds for perceiving it as the basis for shaping individual attachment as well. In the model proposed by Yap et al., (2019) both the biological response of the organism and the internal working models of attachment, moderated by the cultural base, are included in the process of activating the attachment pattern in a cultural context. Thus, the described process resembles the process described by the founders of the basic theory of attachment. It, therefore, seems that attachment is not a personal, internalized, but rather a psychosocial competence. A comprehensive, broader understanding of the child's attachment type or attachment style in adults also resonates with the perspective of the hybrid way of functioning of today's man. The open question is how the accelerating technological changes occurring in specific breakthroughs will influence the shaping of what is called a safe base. What is also extremely interesting is the "whether" and "how" the tendency to attachment, established in successive generations, is realized in a specific way in the online space of contemporary human functioning.

E-attachment: From offline to online

The technology development has changed human development. He expanded the range of possibilities for communication, establishing relationships and finally implementing a social touch in the digital space. Knowledge about the concepts of attachment is available on the Internet. There are screening questionnaires for self-assessment in terms of attachment styles, as well as online courses, workshops and trainings supporting your own work on difficulties resulting from manifesting insecure forms of attachment.

The construct of attachment has received many analyzes and descriptions. The perspectives of several dozen researchers and theorists collected by the team of Thompson et al., (2022) indicate that it is still a complex construct, variously understood, broadly defined and, in principle, differently studied depending on the goal and the studied group. There is a certain consensus that the important element of attachment, which are internal work models, are dynamic structures, changing in the course of development based on successive relational experiences. Despite the cultural diversity, and above all culturally conditioned, different ways of responsiveness, flexibility and accessibility in relation with the other world, it also seems indisputable that attachment is formed in early childhood. It begins with the baby's experiences in contact with its closest caregiver. Consequently, attachment relationships arise in different circumstances and begin to involve other people or objects. As indicated by Thompson et al., (2022) it is, therefore, clear that attachment is one of the fundamental tasks in the course of development.

It is noteworthy that regardless of the differences in the understanding of attachment, the concept of this construct is gaining popularity from time to time both in the world of clinical practitioners and researchers dealing with the development, diagnosis and treatment of mental problems and disorders. Most considerations emphasize the importance of internal working models of attachment and the ways of shaping them (Thompson et al., 2022; Yap et al., 2019; Hong et al., 2013). These, in turn, as already discussed above, are modified by socio-cultural factors.

Understanding the shape of attachment in contemporary reality, with the widespread use of ICT achievements, it seems important to understand what is happening in relationships shaped in the online space. One of the earlier analyzes, conducted by Ye (2007) in a group of over one hundred adults, showed a relationship between the depth of the relationship and satisfaction with it. Analyzing the results of his research, Ye suggested that if people enter into online relationships "to a higher level", they achieve a high level of closeness and comfort regardless of the attachment style presented. This, however, is important in the case of more superficial relationships (in casual relationships). Ye (2007) pointed out that among people with different attachment styles, people with dismissing attachment style are most likely the most satisfied in casual relationships.

It is worth noting, that with the advancement of technology, the spread of media and social networking sites, video games, podcasts, wearables, there is also an option to contact virtual objects. What's more, there is also the possibility of creating virtual characters or digital objects. Is it possible to become attached to this type of object, since as people, we show attachment to culture, surroundings, objects symbolizing our memories and experiences?

Quackenbush et al., (2015) came to interesting conclusions in this regard. Their research among online users showed that attachment can be shaped equally strongly in the real world and in the virtual world. In both cases, they observed a relationship between the duration of the relationship with the object and the strength of attachment. Emotional well-being turned out to correlate with the strength of attachment in the real world, and at the same time with a lower attachment anxiety in the virtual world. Moreover, the researchers indicated that attachment strength in the virtual world is dependent on the ability to fantasize.

The question naturally arises whether attachment in the virtual world is created in parallel or as a result of shaping attachment in the real world. An analysis of known theories of attachment would suggest that working models developed in the early period of life in direct contact with a significant person, constituting a specific backbone of attachment types, de facto constitute a specific pattern that is transferred to later relationships, including virtual ones. Such conclusions were reached in their research by Schönbrodt and Asendorpf (2012).

When analyzing people's decisions regarding virtual relationships, they noticed a convergence between their attachment style and their behavior towards virtual relationship. This trend is also adopted in other studies and is being transferred to clinical experience. In principle, it is not discussed with the assumption whether attachment and its components in reality online are derivative of those from the real world, but rather such an assumption is made from above. Consequently, most research has focused on determining how online functions function in terms of offline attachment (Chicchi Giglioli et al., 2017; Costanzo et al., 2021; Stöven and Herzberg, 2021). However, is such an assumption justified? Observations carried out by Simon (2020), as part of Msc thesis, in a group of several dozen volunteers, users of digital games, showed that, although the presented attachment style is being transferred to virtuality. However, it is not clear what factors are responsible for this transfer. A more complex model of understanding attachment taking place in the virtual world was proposed by Koles and Nagy (2021). Researchers suggested that digital objects should be treated as a broad category, depending on the degree of complexity, user control, interactivity, with value and user meaning. In this sense, a person has contact with digital objects almost constantly, from reading an e-book, through a virtual visit to a museum, searching for virtual pokemons in the space, ending with contact with avatars representing the embodied self of the user in the online space. Koles and Nagy (2021) assume that the process of attachment to virtual objects is possible. The question, then, not "if" but "how" is at the center of their considerations. In their opinion, this process begins with the so-called user dedication. In the initial stage, it is focused on getting to know the possibilities and rules, rules (so-called material culture) prevailing in the virtual space. A person moving for example in an online game must also learn to acquire or create objects and situations, gain knowledge about the functioning and development of their skills in virtual reality. It not only begins to purchase digital goods but also to produce them. Stories are created around them, personal stories that show their meaning, beginnings and fate. In the opinion of Koles and Nagy (2021), these narratives somehow establish an attachment relationship. As a consequence, the process referred to by researchers as psychological ownership is developing. The feeling of belonging to digital objects is manifested by assigning them various features and functions, which is particularly strongly present in the personalization of virtual objects such as avatars. This kind of "appropriation" encourages passion, authority and further personalization of the created reality. The creation of goods and elements with which you can identify allows you to locate yourself in a virtual community. It comes to self-extension. Virtual objects start to live in the world of fantasy and imagination, also when the user is offline. Over time, they can become the basis of experiences used to cope with the real world (transitional properties). The experience of secure attachment, for example related to success, begins to form the basis for coping with emotions or crises experienced in the real world. A mutual dependency relationship arises between transitional properties and object attachment. Koles and Nagy (2021) thus describe two ways of reaching an object attachment – direct and indirect. They assume that they appear cyclically. The second form, through transitional properties, in their opinion, favors the blurring of the boundaries between offline and online.

The concept of an indirect path of development of attachment, especially transitional properties, in a way resembles the concept of transactional objects by Winnicott (1953). In the model proposed by Koles and Nagy (2021), however, the transactional property is a component that lasts. It is not temporary; it does not disappear with the internalization of the virtual object. Instead, it is an element (step) in the process of creating an attachment in the virtual world. In this sense, attachment taking place in virtual reality is in fact a dynamic structure that is constantly being transformed. What's more, a structure that is created at the interface of both realities and not separately in the online and offline world.

Such an approach is consistent with the observations about the changes that modern man undergoes. Assuming further, intensive development of technology, digital touch, and as a consequence of human hybridization, attachment ceases to take place in parallel in two worlds – offline and online. The distinction between these two worlds seems to be justified in relation to that part of the generations that during the first years of their lives developed their self, awareness and attachment in direct, physical contact with objects. This group also includes the authors of this book and, in fact, the vast majority of the research authors cited. There are also many research beliefs that treat virtual reality in a pejorative way. People who engage intensively in the online world are perceived as excessively dreamy, fantasizing in a non-adaptive way in reality, with an insecure attachment style (Costanzo et al., 2021). Meanwhile, the virtual reality that this book partially relates to is evolving all the time. It is a natural and permanent element in the development of children, adolescents and young people who are now entering adulthood. Involvement in the virtual world helps to reduce tension or regulate emotions. The complexity and continuous expansion of the virtual world increase the immersion (level of involvement) in what is virtual, including the relationships taking place in it. For this reason, the virtual world often becomes a place to satisfy emotional needs and build relationships with others. At the same time, it is not only an element of creation, an extension of a human being, but also a part of a human who develops in it. For example, digital technology is present in the fetal stage. Subsequent methods of ultrasound diagnosis modalities (2D, 3D, 4D) allow you to experience yourself in the relationship more and more tangibly during fetal life.

Studies do not show differences in parental attachment depending on the advancement of the ultrasound technology used (Atluru et al., 2012; Benzie et al., 2018). However, the very inclusion of ultrasound technology is considered as one that may directly promote attachment in the womb, or indirectly affect the bond between the mother and the child, by influencing emotions or maternal attitudes (Atluru et al., 2012; Denbow, 2019).

Therefore, modern man interacts with technology before he is able to fully consciously use it. As a consequence, it can be assumed that the "extended" man in this way shapes and activates his potential in one interpenetrating, dynamic, hybrid offline-online space. A space that ceases to be a simple sum of two worlds – the real and the virtual. Such an assumption is in line with a holistic understanding and approach to health and disease – an approach that allows for new trends in the process of thinking about building attachment. A different human structure is created, in which what "E" (related to electronic media) ceases to be just a simple addition, an extension of the individual's boundaries. Assuming that this applies to all human competences, it should also apply to the ability to "attach to", and consequently the attachment itself. This construct is being redefined in a sense. An attempt to capture this change is shown in Figure 2.1. Its symbol is the concept of E–attachment, to emphasize the greater complexity of this construct in relation to traditional descriptions of attachment, and at the same time to distinguish its new, more than extended dimension.

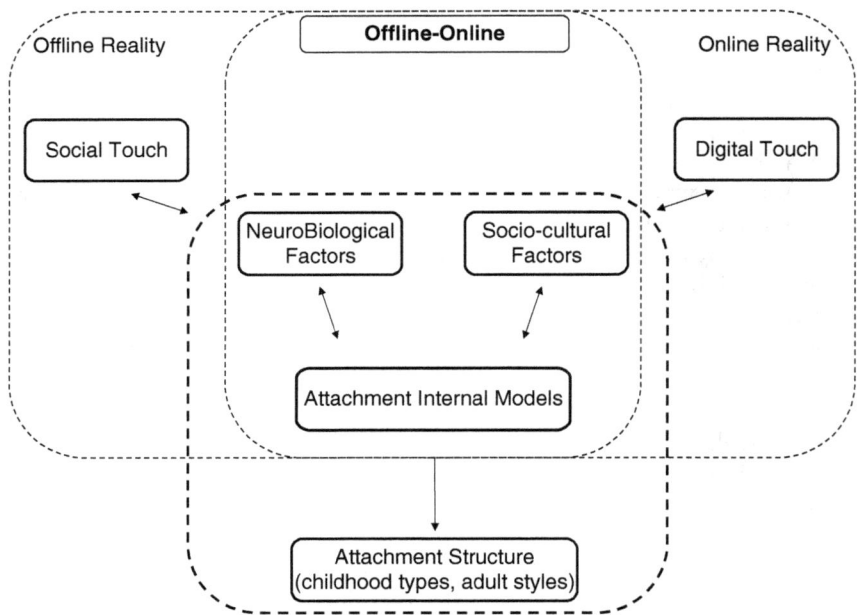

Figure 2.1 E-attachment model proposal.

The assumption that contemporary attachment is shaped in the connected offline-online reality suggests that research focused on observing how attachment patterns formed in direct contact are transferred to the virtual world turns out to be insufficient. E-attachment is a controversial concept, but introduced for reflection on the phenomenon of attachment in the context of a specific revolution that man is undergoing through the increasingly intense development of ITC. Perhaps it is worth returning to the question of whether the currently observed attachment is actually a transfer of the pattern from the real world. How and where are the different aspects of attachment shaped? Does shaping a human being from the first moments of life in a reality using modern technologies give rise to assuming that the character and method of forming an attachment change? Are the current theories of attachment sufficient to understand what is happening with attachment at the offline-online level? These are the questions that constitute the starting point for research in the field of attachment in the modern world.

References

Ainsworth, M.D.S. (2021). Attachment. In: T. Forslund, R. Duschinsky, *Attachment Theory and Research* (pp. 46–73). New York: Wiley-Blackwell.

Ainsworth, M.D.S., Bowlby, J. (1991). An ethological approach to personality development. *American Psychologist*, 46(4), 333–341. DOI: 10.1037/0003-066X.46.4.333

Atluru, A., Appleton, K., Plavsic, S. (2012). Maternal-Fetal Bonding: Ultrasound Imaging's Role in enhancing This Important Relationship. *Donald School Journal of Ultrasound in Obstetrics and Gynecology*, 6, 408–411. DOI: 10.5005/jp-journals-10009-1263

Bartholomew, K., Shaver, P.R. (1998). Methods of assessing adult attachment. Do they converge? In: J. A. Simpson, W. S. Rholes (Eds.), *Attachment Theory and Close Relationships* (pp. 24–45) New York: Guilford Press.

Benoit, D. (2004). Infant-parent attachment: Definition, types, antecedents, measurement and outcome. *Pediatrics & Child Health*, 9(8), 541–545. DOI: 10.1093/pch/9.8.541

Benzie, R.J., Starcevic, V., Viswasam, K., Kennedy, N.J., Mein, B.J., Wye, D.A., Martin, A. (2018). Effect of three- vs four-dimensional ultrasonography on maternal attachment. *Ultrasound in Obstetrics Gynecology*, 51(4), 558–559. DOI: 10.1002/uog.17567

Bowlby, J. (2021). *Przywiązanie*. Warszawa: PWN.

Bretherton, I. (1992). The origins of attachment theory: John Bowlby and Mary Ainsworth. *Developmental Psychology*, 28, 759–775. DOI: https://doi.org/10.1037/0012-1649.28.5.759

Chicchi Giglioli, I. A., Pravettoni, G., Sutil, M.D.L., Parra, E., Raya, M.A. (2017). A Novel Integrating Virtual Reality Approach for the Assessment of the Attachment Behavioral System.*Frontiers in Psychology*, 8, 959. DOI: 10.3389/fpsyg.2017.00959

Costanzo, A., Santoro, G., Russo, S., Cassarà, M.S., Midolo, L.R., Billieux, J., Schimmenti, A. (2021). Attached to Virtual Dreams: The Mediating Role of Maladaptive Daydreaming in the Relationship Between Attachment Styles and Problematic Social Media Use. *Journal of Nervous and Mental Disease*, 209(9), 656–664. DOI: 10.1097/NMD.0000000000001356

Denbow, J. (2019). Good Mothering Before Birth: Measuring Attachment and Ultrasound as an Affective Technology. *Engaging Science, Technology, and Society*, 5, 1–20. DOI: 10.1 7351/ests2019.238

Duschinsky, R. (2018). Disorganization, fear and attachment: working towards clarification. *Infant Mental Health Journal*, 39(1), 17–29. DOI: 10.1002/imhj.21689

Eder, S.J., Nicholson, A.A., Stefanczyk, M.M., Pieniak, M., Martínez-Molina, J., Pešout, O., Binter, J., Smela, P., Scharnowski, F., Steyrl, D. (2021). Securing Your Relationship: Quality of Intimate Relationships During the COVID-19 Pandemic Can Be Predicted by Attachment Style. *Frontiers in Psychology*, 12, 647956. DOI: 10.3389/fpsyg.2021.647956

Granqvist, P. (2021). Attachment, culture, and gene-culture co-evolution: expanding the evolutionary toolbox of attachment theory. *Attachment & Human Development*, 23(1), 90–113. 10.1080/14616734.2019.1709086

Granqvist, P., Sroufe, L.A., Dozier, M., Hesse, E., Steele, M., van Ijzendoorn, M., Steele, H. (2017). Disorganized attachment in infancy: A review of the phenomenon and its implications for clinicians and policy-makers. *Attachment & Human Development*, 19(6), 534–558. DOI: 10.1111/jir.12217

Harlow, H.F. (1958). The nature of love. *American Psychologist*, 13(12), 673–685. DOI: 10.1 037/h0047884

Hong, Y., Fang, Y., Yang, Y., Phua, D.Y. (2013). Cultural Attachment: A New Theory and Method to Understand Cross-Cultural Competence. *Journal of Cross-Cultural Psychology*, 44(6), 1024–1044. DOI: 10.1177/0022022113480039

Koles, B., Nagy, P. (2021). Digital object attachment. *Current Opinion in Psychology*, 39, 60–65. DOI: 10.1016/j.copsyc.2020.07.017

Main, M., Solomon, J. (1986). Discovery of an insecure-disorganized/disoriented attachment pattern. In: T. B. Brazelton, M. W. Yogman. *Affective Development in Infancy* (pp. 95–124). Norwood: Ablex.

Mesman, J., van IJzendoorn, M.H., Sagi-Schartz, A. (2016). Cross-cultural patterns of attachment: Universal and contextual dimensions. In: J. Cassidy, P. R. Shaver, (eds.) *Handbook of Attachment: Theory, Research, and Clinical Applications*. 3. (pp. 852–877). New York: Guilford Press.

Mikulincer, M., Shaver, P.R., Pereg, D. (2003). Attachment Theory and Affect Regulation: The Dynamics, Development, and Cognitive Consequences of Attachment-Related Strategies. *Motivation and Emotion*, 27, 77–102. DOI: 10.1023/A:1024515519160

Mikulincer, M., Shaver, P. R. (2016). *Attachment in Adulthood: Structure, Dynamics, and Change* (2nd ed.). New York, NY: Guilford Press.

Morales-Vives, F., Ferré-Rey, G., Ferrando, P.J., Camps, M. (2021). Balancing typological and dimensional approaches: Assessment of adult attachment styles with Factor Mixture Analysis. *PLoS ONE*, 16(7). DOI: 10.1371/journal.pone.0254342

Opie, J.E., McIntosh, J.E., Esler, T.B., Duschinsky, R., George, C., Schore, A., Kothe, E.J., Tan, E.S., Greenwood C.J., Olsson C.A. (2021). Early childhood attachment stability and change: a meta-analysis, *Attachment & Human Development*, 23(6), 897–930. DOI: 10.1080/14616734.2020.1800769

Parsons, T.D. (2017). *Cyberpsychology and the Brain: The Interaction of Neuroscience and Affective Computing* (p. 409). Cambridge University Press. Kindle Edition.

Pilkonis, P.A., Kim, Y., Yu, L., Morse, J.Q. (2013). Adult Attachment Ratings (AAR): An Item Response Theory Analysis. *Journal of Personality Assessment*, 96(4), 417–425. DOI: 10.1080/00223891.2013.832261

Prensky, M. (2001). Digital natives, digital immigrants part 1. *On the Horizon*, 9, 1–6.

Pritchard, A.E., Kalback, S., Capone G.T. (2015). Executive functions among youth with Down syndrome and co-existing neurobehavioural disorders. *Journal of Intellectual Disability Research*, 59(12), 1130–1141. DOI: 10.1111/jir.12217

Quackenbush, D., Allen, J.G., Fowler, J.C. (2015). Comparison of Attachments in Real-World and Virtual-World Relationships. *Psychiatry*, 78(4), 317–327. DOI: 10.1080/00332747.2015.1092854

Rothbaum, F., Weisz, J., Pott, M., Miyake, K., Morelli, G. (2000). Attachment and culture.Security in the United States and Japan. *American Psychology*, 55(10), 1093–1104. DOI: 10.1037//0003-066x.55.10.1093

Schönbrodt, F.D., Asendorpf, J.B. (2012). Attachment dynamics in a virtual world. *Journal of Personalized Medicine*, 80(2), 429–463. DOI: 10.1111/j.1467-6494.2011.00736.x

Simon, W. (2020). *Virtual Attachment: How Attachment Styles Transfer into Virtuality*. Master's thesis presented to the Department of Psychology of the University of Basel for the degree of Master of Science in Psychology. https://www.mmi-basel.ch/MA/2020_Wehrli.pdf

Stein, H., Koontz, A.D., Fonagy, P., Allen, J.G., Fultz, J., Brethour, J.R. (2002). Adult attachment: What are the underlying dimensions? *Psychology and Psychotherapy: Theory, Research and Practice*, 75, 77–91. DOI: 10.1348/147608302169562

Stöven, L.M., Herzberg, P.Y. (2021). Relationship 2.0: A systematic review of associations between the use of social network sites and attachment style. *Journal of Social and Personal Relationships*, 38(3), 1103–1128. DOI: 10.1177/0265407520982671

Strand, P.S., Vossen, J.J., & Savage, E. (2019). Culture and Child Attachment Patterns: a Behavioral Systems Synthesis. *Perspectives on behavior science*, 42(4), 835–850. DOI: 10.1007/s40614-019-00220-3

Thompson, R.A., Simpson, J.A., Berlin, L.J. (2022). Taking perspective on attachment theory and research: nine fundamental questions. *Attachment and Human Development*, 24, 1–18. DOI: 10.1080/14616734.2022.2030132

Vanwalleghem, S., Miljkovitch, R., Vinter, A. (2021). Attachment representations among school-age children with intellectual disability. *Research in Developmental Disabilities*, 118, 104064. DOI: 10.1016/j.ridd.2021.10406

Winnicott, D.W. (1953). Transitional objects and transitional phenomena; a study of the first not-me possession. *The International Journal of Psychoanalysis*, 34(2), 89–97.

Yap, W.J., Cheon, B., Hong, Y.Y., Christopoulos, G.I. (2019). Cultural Attachment: From Behavior to Computational Neuroscience. *Frontiers in Human Neuroscience*, 13, 1–17. DOI: 10.3389/fnhum.2019.00209

Ye, J. (2007). Attachment style differences in online relationship involvement: An examination of interaction characteristics and relationship satisfaction. *CyberPsychology & Behavior*, 10(4), 605–607. DOI: 10.1089/cpb.2007.9982

Chapter 3

Attachment, relationships and new technologies from a neuroscience perspective

Chapter overview

The aim of this chapter is to answer the question whether the neural and physiological correlates of bonding and interpersonal relationships are the same in online interactions as in face-to-face interactions. The first part of the chapter provides a selective overview of the neurobiological correlates of attachment theory for language reconciliation and a starting point for further analysis. Then, selected theses of social neuroscience are described, showing the possibility of dynamics and interaction of various neural circuits in interpersonal situations. The main part of the chapter describes the neural and physiological issues related to building an online therapeutic relationship and relationship between the patient and the specialist. Finally, the slightly wider context is described – the functioning of the brain when building relationships in the online environment, including social networks. Hypotheses and speculations are quite frequent in the text, as the research base on the topics discussed here is still limited, and the reports so far are ambiguous.

Brain and new technologies

Probably no one is surprised that the brain is called a social organ, meaning that every social interaction is reflected in neurobiological systems, and more importantly, the brain shows a remarkable motivation to seek and interact with other people. Previous studies on diagnosis, psychological help and psychotherapy show that establishing relationships with others carries a healing potential, modifying behavior or influencing the internal mental states of an individual, which is the main topic in the pages of this book. Perhaps the analysis of interpersonal phenomena from the neurobiological point of view will bring us closer to the answer to the question about the similarity of the face-to-face relationship to the one created online, called e-attachment in this book. So the purpose of this chapter is to review the selected literature and reflect on the question – do internet relationships engage the brain in the same way as real-world interactions? Certain reservations should be made in the

DOI: 10.4324/9781003221043-4

introduction: first of all, this chapter is not a comprehensive compendium of neuroscience or a text for neuropsychology specialists, but rather a review of basic knowledge and a free and sometimes speculative reflection on the biological correlates of interpersonal relations. The word "speculative" comes up because there are still many questions and unresolved hypotheses waiting to be solved in the area described here. Second, we intentionally quote very rarely in this chapter, and sometimes completely omit research on animals, not because it is unimportant but because it clearly exceeds the substantive and, above all, volumetric framework of this chapter. Third, it is especially important for people less familiar with the knowledge of the brain – it is in vain to look for simple solutions that a single place in the brain corresponds to human behavior, or rather we can talk about structural and functional networks influencing each other in a complex way. In the first part of the chapter, we will focus on a basic overview of knowledge about the neurobiological foundations of the theory of attachment, in the second part, we will try to relate to these correlates in the context of online interpersonal interactions.

Attachment Theory

To begin with, let's look at the basic knowledge of neurobiological functioning in the context of interpersonal relationships. Attachment theory was strongly rooted in ethology and biology from the outset, through the work of its pioneer John Bowlby. He described how important an evolutionary element is for a human being to have a close bond with the caregiver because they were unable to cope without one. It is a specific instinct of a two-sided nature: on the one hand, the child strives for the caregiver, calls him back, and on the other hand, the guardian shows motivation to take care of the child, which, according to evolutionary theories, gives the best chance of maintaining the transferred gene pool (Bowlby, 1969; Buss, 2019). And this is not only a relationship based on the technical satisfaction of physiological and nutritional needs, as evidence was first provided by Harlow (Seay and Harlow, 1965) in his monkey studies, but also largely related to emotional regulation and dealing with developmental propositions. Thus, a specific interaction between the child and psychosocial attachment figures arises, supported by biological and neurocognitive structures and mechanisms. Are we able to identify them?

As mentioned in the introduction, in order to interact or even interact closely with others, a person and his brain must have the motivation to initiate and sustain such activities. Probably evolutionarily it is very justified, because a man cannot cope independently without the help of a guardian, for a very long time, going well beyond the infancy period. Thus, in order for the human species to survive, it had to develop mechanisms for the efforts of the child and the guardian to get together. Moreover, working in cooperation with others also in adulthood has brought people as a species many benefits, not only in mutual support of partners, in raising children, but also in loyal cooperation of whole groups and communities, thanks to which our species has mastered the earth like no other.

The reward system probably plays a very important role in this motivation and initiation of interpersonal interactions. It includes the dopamine projection system of the ventral tegmental area and substantia nigra which project dopamine into various discrete sites and neural networks, in particular the nucleus accumbens.

Research has shown that with the activation of the ventral tegmental area and the nucleus accumbens, there is a feeling of pleasure and the strengthening of certain behaviors, not only in the real situation but also in the situation of anticipated reward. It has been proven that dopaminergic neurons in the ventral tegmental area become sensitive over time to primarily unconditioned stimuli, including those of a social nature. This sequence is the neural equivalent of the conditioning situation and the reinforcement of goal-directed behavior. (J. Coan, 2019; Lammel et al., 2014). Dopamine deficiencies, experimentally induced in animals by damage to the ventral tegmental area or nucleus accumbens, reduce or eliminate the caring behavior of the rat mother, while maintaining other functions, such as nest building or passive feeding (Hansen et al., 1991).

It also seems that the neuropeptides oxytocin and vasopressin play a very important role in attachment behavior (Morrone-Strupinsky and Depue, 2005; Young and Wang, 2004). Both are related to the shaping of the partner's preferences and the pursuit of him regardless of mating behavior. Both of these substances, especially oxytocin, can be triggered by positive social behavior (Carter, 2014). In response to social signals, oxytocin and vasopressin enhance the dopaminergic activity in the ventral tegmental area and in the nucleus accumbens (Shahrokh et al., 2010). In prairie voles, known for their monogamous, long-term bonding in pairs and cooperation in various aspects of functioning (nesting, defense of the territory, caring for young), it has been observed that the nucleus accumbens is extremely rich in oxytocin receptors, and the ventral tegmental area and abdominal globe pale they are rich in vasopressin receptors. Such rich receptors have not been observed in non-monogamous animals, including other varieties of voles (Carter et al., 1995; Insel and Fernald, 2004; Lim and Young, 2006; Young and Wang, 2004). Therefore, there is probably a feedback loop in which oxytocin and vasopressin are released in response to social interactions, which in turn stimulate the dopaminergic system, which, as described above, is associated with the feeling of pleasure and strengthening a specific behavior (in this case, entering into social interactions and the search for closeness).

Another important structure of the brain in the context of attachment may be the amygdala. One of the best-known longitudinal studies showed that people with an insecure attachment pattern tested at 18 months of age, at 22 years of age, had more amygdala volume compared to people with a secure attachment pattern (Moutsiana et al., 2015). There was no such correlation in these studies with the hippocampus. Similar research (Lyons-Ruth et al., 2016) showed that people who presented desorganized attachemnt in early childhood in the Strange Situation Procedure and their mothers communicated incorrectly at the age of 29 also had an enlarged body almond-shaped, especially on the left side. Later stressors, for example in adolescence, had no effect on changes in the volume of amygdala. So here we see a special meaning of amygdala in the context of attachment. It is probably related to many important human functions that make up all human interactions. For example, perhaps Amygdala is directly related to facial recognition (Benuzzi et al., 2007; Rolls, 2007), and above all, to emotions (Johansen et al., 2011). People with amygdala dysfunction have difficulty processing emotional facial expressions, especially those of social importance, while in healthy people, the facial expressions of others properly activate the amygdala.

In the context of attachment, memory in a broad sense is also very important – people, including babies, must remember their relatives, recognize them, associate them with the external context and internal states. Here, the amygdala and the hippocampus probably also play an extremely important role, including the creation, storage and consolidation of stimuli, internal states and the environmental context. Research has shown that amygdala activity during the information encoding phase is associated with recalling emotionally relevant information several weeks later (Hamann et al., 1999).

Although the research is inconclusive in this area, the hypothalamic-pituitary-adrenal axis (HPA) probably plays a role in attachment interactions. The first of these elements – the hypothalamus connects the nervous and endocrine systems and regulates various autonomic and metabolic processes. It is likely that the hypothalamus receives information related to social situations, emotions, attachment or stress from various brain structures (e.g. the amygdala, hippocampus, prefrontal cortex), and then releases the corticotropin stimulating hormone (CRH) in response to this, and this attracts a number of further reactions, for example the release of adenocorticotropic hormone (ACTH), the production of cortisol and adrenaline, affect the subjective perception of stress and agitation, or norepinephrine. In several studies, children who displayed an insecure attachment responded with higher levels of cortisol in response to separation and other stressors, compared to children displaying a secure bond (Ahnert et al., 2004). In other studies, in turn, secure children showed significant increases in their cortisol levels after fear episodes and significant decreases, after positive affect ones. In children with insecure attachment no changes in cortisol were noted, hence the researchers speculated that in this group there may be inhibition of the HPA axis (insecure attachment may be related to hypothalamic-pituitary-adrenal axis suppression in response to challenging and positive contexts).

Another important structure of the brain that is possibly coordinating and involved in the emotional regulation of social interaction and attachment is the hypothalamus. The hypothalamus likely coordinates the activity of many behavioral and physiological systems, including those involved in maternal behavior and pairing, although the detailed mechanisms are yet to be understood (J. A. Coan et al., 2006; Conner et al., 2012; Kim and Kochanska, 2015).

At the very top of the evolutionary ladder is the prefrontal cortex, which is believed to be a very important factor in emotional regulation. The prefrontal cortex is strongly connected to the dopaminergic projection system (e.g. nucleus accumbens and ventral tegmental area), the amygdala, hippocampus and hypothalamus. Moreover, it is believed that ventromedial and medial orbital prefrontal cortex are likely to be responsible for the automatic regulation of emotions, and dorsolateral prefrontal cortex to be volitional, that is responsible for the use of attention, working memory and other complex cognitive functions. Thus, it is believed that the prefrontal cortex can respond to attachment processes in two ways: automatic responses to the attachment figure in response to a threat signal and cognitive operations regarding attachment figures in working memory (Ochsner et al., 2012). Prefrontal cortex also plays a role in interpersonal emotional regulation. In animal models, it was found that two rats subjected to a stressful situation reduce each other's stress levels (Lungwitz et al., 2014). It probably also happens in the situation of psychotherapy – a patient who tells the therapist about difficult and stressful life events uses the therapeutic relationship to regulate the tension resulting from recalling these situations (Chambers, 2017). The role of interpersonal relations and their neural correlates in the regulation of emotions is the main area of interest for the so-called social neuroscience as will be discussed below.

The medial prefrontal cortex, the bilateral temporo-parietal junction, the upper temporal furrow, preclinics and temporal poles are possibly key to theorizing about the minds of others, and what has been called theory of mind and mentalization in psychology (Kovács et al., 2014). These functions are very important because they strongly influence relationship building, emotional regulation and many other functions, and abnormalities in this area are probably a component of many disorders, for example some personality disorders or autism spectrum disorders (Frith and Frith, 2003; Saxe and Kanwisher, 2003).

The last of the most important elements is the mirror neurons system, which was first discovered in monkeys by Rizzolatti et al. (Rizzolatti et al., 1996). Initially, it was postulated that this system is responsible for recognizing, understanding and imitating others. Even though a monkey or a human does not perform a given activity but observes it in another individual, these neural networks are activated in their brains. With subsequent publications, these neurons were assigned more and more importance, going much further beyond simple imitation, for example empathy towards others, understanding internal states and intentions of other people, etc. Structurally, the mirror neurons system covers the posterior part of the inferior frontal gyrus, the ventral part of the cortex premotor, superior temporal furrow, anterior part of the island, amygdala, premotor cortex and inferior parietal lobe.

All the above-described areas do not work in isolation, but they cooperate with each other in various and complicated ways in the context of interpersonal relations, and the manner of this cooperation can be interpreted in various ways. Let us take the following example showing the sequence of events in the nervous system in response to a hypothetical event – meeting an attractive partner: (1) meeting with an attractive partner results in the release of dopamine from the ventral tegmental area, which stimulates dopaminergic activity in the nucleus accumbens related to the feeling of pleasure, including anticipatory. (2) The amygdala indicates the sensory properties of the stimulus (partner) as important from an individual point of view during the process of consolidating long-term memory through (3) the hippocampus, which at the same time encodes contextual information of the stimulus (what circumstances accompany the meeting, is the partner also interested in us, etc.). Prefrontal cortex integrates and uses this information to create and implement action plans related to this stimulus (what will happen in the current situation and other anticipated situations, including what benefits may result from meeting a partner). These elements will increase the willingness and likelihood of another meeting with a partner and the feedback loop strengthens the beginning of the sequence, that is activation of the dopaminergic system. A similar pattern can be imagined in the case of motivation to move away and in any other relationship in which the person anticipates benefits for himself on various levels: biological, social, emotional (e.g. when meeting a therapist to solve his own problems) (Zeifman and Hazan, 1997).

Social neuroscience

The anatomical and physiological correlates presented above are, in a way, scattered blocks. The field that tries to combine these elements with each other, recognizing the interrelationships between the real social behavior of a person and the functioning of the brain is Social neuroscience. Within this domain, various sub-models are developed that cannot all be covered in this section. For example, we will present one of them, called a comprehensive functional neuro-anatomical model of human attachment (NAMA). It should be added that this is a hypothetical model within which the existing research data that directly or indirectly concerns attachment has been collected.

NAMA model

The NAMA model (White et al., 2020) assumes that due to the need to adapt to the environment and return to homeostasis, there are two neurobiological systems driving this process: the affective-emotional system and the cognitive control system. Further, each of them consists of two modules:

* as part of the affective emotional system, we have a module called aversion negative module, coding social events such as a threat or abandonment.

An important element in this module will be the basic stress hormone, that is cortisol, acting through the HPA axis,

- at the same time, the stress or fear reaction triggers a second module called the approach module triggers the regulation response by "escaping towards another person" (attachemnt figure) because probably social relations are coded at the neuronal level as internally rewarding and at the neuronal level it will be associated with the reward system and hormones such as oxytocin and dopamine or vasopressin, which we also wrote about in the previous section.

Both of these modules are activated by, and represent more automatic, bottom-up and specified as affective evaluation or emotional mentalization processes. They are relatively independent and complementary at the same time, and can be hyperactivated or deactivated in a variety of attachment-relevant situations.

After establishing the motivation to look for others in the affective emotional system as a source of emotional regulation and social support, the next stage may take place within the second system: the cognitive control system, which also consists of two modules: (1) emotional (self-) regulation module where emotion regulation takes place, in two ways – outside through "co-regulation" in the presence of others or as self-regulation as a result of internalization of significant attachment figures. The neural correlates of this module will likely be located in the dorsolateral prefrontal cortex; and lateral orbitofrontal cortex. The second module included in the cognitive control system is (2) mental state representation module, can be understood according to the NAMA model as an equivalent of internal working models, which is created as a result of repeated interactions with other people, and includes predictions as to when and who is in need and who and when will be beneficial in such situations. The neural counterparts of this module will likely be located in the medial prefrontal cortex; posterior cingulate cortex/precuneus, posterior superior temporal sulcus/temporo-parietal junction, anterior superior temporal, gyrus, fusiform gyrus. The emotional (self-) regulation and mental state representation modules are part of the cognitive/control system and rather associated with top-down regulation.

It should be noted that the above description is for a prototype adaptive attachment. It can be added that it differs from insecure attachment in general in the greater integrity of the aversion module along with the HPA axis. In turn, it is presumed that avoidant attachment is more related to the decreased functionality of the approach module, including for example reduced amounts of oxytocin and opioids, making interpersonal relationships less pleasant and satisfying. In turn, anxious-ambivalent attachment will be more closely related to the activation of the aversion module, in particular the HPA axis activation, and then the persistence of this increased activation (unavailability of cognitive/control system adjustment.

A separate issue is to identify the neural correlates of disorganized attachment, that is the one that, according to research, is most often associated with early neglect, abuse, abuse or other early childhood traumas. Some studies have demonstrated the hyperactivity of the HPA system and the associated higher levels of cortisol (Bernard and Dozier, 2010; Hertsgaard et al., 1995; Spangler and Grossmann, 1993), which would suggest that people with disorganized attachment show the highest HPA reactivity. However, other large studies have not confirmed this hypothesis, showing that the highest activity of the HPA system is presented by people classified as anxious–ambivalent (Luijk et al., 2010; Spangler and Schieche, 1998). However, there is some heterogeneity in the research methodology, for example in one of the above-cited studies, the shortened Strange Situation Procedure was used, which could lead to differences in classifying children to particular patterns of attachment. In addition, there are also studies that show a different trend, namely a flattening of the cortisol curve over the course of the day and a constant "suppression" of cortisol levels (Luijk et al., 2010; Reilly and Gunnar, 2019; Schalinski et al., 2019; White et al., 2017). It is presumed that this may be the result of internal (biological) self-regulation, which at the same time makes regulation independent of other people at the behavioral level. Other studies indicate the probable role of the amygdala, both its increased activation (Buchheim et al., 2006, 2008) and its volume, both in human and animal studies (Howell et al., 2014; Lupien et al., 2011; Lyons–Ruth et al., 2016; Mehta et al., 2009; Moutsiana et al., 2015), which would explain the constant fear and freeze in reaction to the caregiver. As mentioned earlier, the above model was presented as an example, but there are also other known models in the literature that try to explain the issues raised here (Callaghan and Tottenham, 2016; Humphreys and Zeanah, 2015; Sheridan and McLaughlin, 2014; Teicher et al., 2016).

Interpersonal neurobiology, on-line psychotherapy and psychotherapeutic relationship

In the process of psychological assistance, especially in psychotherapy, the special role of the therapeutic relationship is emphasized as a factor of key importance for the effectiveness of treatment (Norcross and Lambert, 2018). Based on the attachment theory, it can be stated that in a psychotherapeutic relationship, as in any other interpersonal relationship, a specific bond pattern is activated for each person, which was formed during early interactions with significant people (parents, caregivers). Therefore, many clinicians and theorists agree, however, in creating a relationship with the patient, the behavior of good therapists is in some sense (and even should be) very similar to the behavior of good parents towards their children (Marmarosh et al., 2013; Wallin, 2007). The following few paragraphs will be devoted to these topics in online psychological help, including neurobiological processes.

Psychotherapist vs avatar

Research on psychological help and psychotherapy online, although so far still small compared to face to face, gives promising results both in terms of its effectiveness (Varker et al., 2018; Weinberg and Rolnick, 2019) and the creation of relationships therapeutic (Beintner et al., 2019; Jasper et al., 2014; Pihlaja et al., 2018; Sucala et al., 2012). Building a therapeutic relationship in online psychological help is very specific and diverse – today's technology offers various possibilities when it comes to the form of a specialist during the online diagnosis and help process. A "psychologist or therapist" can be a website, a computer program, or a well-designed Internet forum. It can also be a competent psychologist hiding behind a voice from a telephone without a vision, an icon or an avatar. This may have various consequences for building a therapeutic relationship. To illustrate this phenomenon, one can cite the research on how people, perceiving virtual characters, understand their behavior. The respondents, observing the figures on the computer screen, were to classify whether their movements were natural or artificial. The results showed that the perception of behavior as natural increases with the virtual character more closely resembling a real human – the subjects observed characters ranging from primitive diagrams of dots to fully reflected person in the diagram (Chaminade et al., 2007). The use of fMRI in these studies showed that the perception of movement as natural correlated positively with the activity of the left temporo-parietal junction and anterior cingulate gyrus, that is areas associated with attention control and mentalizing network, while inversely correlated with the activity of areas related to the motor cortex (related to the so-called mirror system). The authors of these studies explain this phenomenon by the need to give meaning to the characters' movements on the screen, and not just to simply reflect these movements. It should be added that the primitive characters on the screen (composed of dots) did not correlate with the activation of areas of the brain. Other studies have also shown activation closely related to the theory of mind, i.e. the upper temporal sulcus, the lateral fusiform gyrus, and the mid-temporal gyrus when interpreting a figure's facial and eye movements on a computer screen (Pelphrey and Carter, 2008).

Thus, a cautious conclusion might be that the psychological support issues related to the need for mentalization will require either "live" participants of online interactions or at least closely human-like avatars. And you can imagine this issue in two directions – not only the specialist seeing his patient, but also the patient seeing the specialist.

Therapeutic relationship and mirror neurons

Interpersonal nuerobiology, using reports on mirror neurons, tries to explain how the process of creating bonds between people, including the patient and the clinician, can be reflected at the neuronal level. The following paragraphs briefly describe this idea.

Once again, we must emphasize that the brain is a social organ, which means that it seeks out other brains, synchronizes with them, learns from them, etc., and the brains constantly change their structure through these interactions. Alan Schore (2014, 2021) and Daniel Siegiel (Siegel, 2007, 2015) emphasize in particular the large role of the right hemisphere in the brain in this respect. This approach takes into account several components. First, there are three cognitive aspects: memory – explicit, implicit and autobiographical. Second, mirror neurons, which are the basis of emotional synchronization and regulation, and third, four domains of neural integration – integration of consciousness, interpersonal, vertical and bilateral integration.

When it comes to autobiographical memory, human brains encode the earliest attachment relationships that are the pattern for future relationships, and most of these memories will be encoded in implicit form. It is an idea similar to that formulated by founders of attachment theory (Bowlby, 1969, 1982; Bretherton and Munholland, 2016), that is the existence of internal working models, which reflect the connections between the attachment figure's proximity and internal needs and signs of external threat, which at the neuronal level probably it happens through the amygdala, nucleus accumbens and hippocampus, as well as parts of the prefrontal cortex. These models can remain stable for a long time, especially to the extent that they are still reinforced by an inner sense of security, prevailing social circumstances, or both.

We also know that conditioned associations can remain stable for a long time, especially to the extent that they are still strengthened by an inner sense of security, prevailing social circumstances, or both (Hofer, 2006). When mirror neurons begin to function, we begin to represent the intentions and feelings of others towards us by coding it in our minds (Iacoboni, 2009b, 2009a). The sensory parts of the neocortex also encode bits of experience – eyes, smell, texture, sound and touch. Our limbic system, especially the amygdala and the right hemisphere in particular, develops neural pathways through experience. When infants interact with their mother in the first 12 to 18 months of life, a special type of memory is formed, but different from the type of memory we know from adult life. These are the memories encoded in the implicit memory, consisting of bodily sensations, behavioral impulses, emotional tides, a sense of security or lack thereof, as well as possible fragmentary images as described above. If these memories are activated in adulthood, they are very often confused with the present reality, intertwined with current life events and are experienced unambiguously as actual, real reality. Later in childhood brain development, connections are formed between the amygdala (the central element of implicit memory) with the hippocampus (responsible for explicit memory), and then with the prefrontal cortex, which enables memory to be integrated into a coherent narrative, that is autobiographical memory. It should be added that traumatic events can disrupt these integration processes by excessive action of neurohormones (Schore, 2003, 2009).

The above processes, and in particular, the discovery of mirror neurons, which are an important element of subliminal interactions with others, made it possible to formulate many new very promising hypotheses about the functioning of the brain in the context of interpersonal relations. The main hypothesis is that mirror neurons align individuals with the possibility of a connection between brains/minds, and supports the claim that the brain is a social organ (Cozolino, 2014). Individuals do not live in social isolation, existing independently next to each other, but rather are constantly interacting with others and reflecting the interpersonal world. There are authors who prove that mirror neurons connect representatives of the same species at the precognitive level, fire in response to specific circumstances – in a situation of goal orientation, the need for empathy, intentional action, also reacting to various stimuli, including social stimuli. signals, body language, gestures, facial expressions, voice, etc. (Iacoboni, 2008). In other words, this idea explains the fact of pre-linguistic communication between mother and child, their mutual reflection and modeling in interpersonal relations, non-verbal interpersonal communication, and finally non-linguistic communication between the patient and the specialist, for example during psychological assistance or psychotherapy.

Thus, a hypothetical model based on the above-mentioned types of memory and mirror neuron networks may give a hypothetical picture of how different interactions may occur within the relationship with a psychologist, psychotherapist or therapeutic group. On the one hand, the nervous circuits related to implicit memory can lead to a number of different expectations of the patient towards the clinician, or attitudes, which in the dynamic approach in psychotherapy are called transference. On the other hand, in the process, when a therapeutic relationship is established, there may be reflection and interbrain synchronization, which contributes to the actual emotional regulation and thus to the formation of a constant pattern of emotional self-regulation. In addition, during the process of diagnosis or psychological support, areas of the brain responsible for the above-described types of memory may be stimulated (e.g. through an interview, telling about life and problems), which causes the patient to experience a wide variety of emotions. The mirror neurons of a calm, empathetic, reflective therapist will resonate with the patient's brain, thus modeling his internal state.

It should be emphasized once again that the role of mirror neurons has not been fully understood, is associated with many uncertainties and, by some, it is also widely criticized. It can be concluded that the models based on the operation of mirror networks are still in the research phase, hence it must be remembered that they cannot be understood definitively, but rather as hypotheses for further research.

Online therapeutic relationship and psychophysiological synchrony

Similarly to the psychophysiological matching between mother and child, it occurs spontaneously, especially with proper bonding between them (Gray et al., 2018; Healey et al., 2010; Woody et al., 2016), then also in the period of adolescents (Li et al., 2020), this is also how such synchronization may occur when building a therapeutic relationship between the therapist and the patient. We describe here physiological and neuronal synchronization, which may refer to such aspects as: stimulation of similar brain centers, skin conductance, specifically cardiac and electrodermal activity, facial myography, skin temperature, respiratory rhythms, speech pitch, etc. (Kleinbub et al., 2020). Sample research in this field showed that physiological synchronization is associated with core positive qualities of the therapist, such as the therapist's empathy (Marci et al., 2007) observed that a stimulus aimed at priming secure attachment increased physiological synchronization and its dynamics in psychotherapists in training and Tourunen et al., (2020) has found that changes in physiological synchronization were related to changes in the therapeutic alliance. Unequivocally settled, however, preliminary data confirm that it may be more difficult in online therapy than in face-to-face therapy. A study by (Jiang et al., 2012) showed that compared to other types of communication, face-to-face communication is characterized by significant neural synchronization between partners (significant increase in neural synchronization in the left lower frontal cortex in face-to-face dialogue but not in other types of communication). According to the authors, this synchronization is based on the multimodal integration of sensory information and the alternating behavior during communication. These results indicate that face-to-face communication has important neural characteristics that other types of communication lack, and that people should spend more time communicating face-to-face.

If there is such a discrepancy, how can it be explained? Let us try to look at some specificity of the work of psychologists and therapists during online sessions with patients. To begin with, it should be said that working online has its undeniable benefits, especially regarding the economy of time and finance, as well as accessibility (Weinberg and Rolnick, 2019). On the other hand, it also has its limitations. Although these issues have not been studied in detail so far, the work of online psychotherapists in personal experience requires greater concentration, observation and processing of other information than in face to face psychotherapy, which ultimately leads to greater psychophysical exhaustion (Marks-Tarlow, 2021; Piasecka et al., 2021) Other inconveniences include the need to have the ability to operate computer hardware and software, watching yourself on the screen during the session (by default, communication programs show all participants of the conversation on the screen) – which redirects a large part of attention to yourself, discovering your own intimacy when therapeutic sessions are conducted with home and the discrepancy in the context of the meeting (previously the therapist and the patient were in the same room and were subjected to the same subliminal stimuli, now the therapist and the patient are in two different external contexts). These factors may make it difficult to build an intimate atmosphere of a meeting, a comprehensive and unambiguous clinical assessment and the aforementioned psychophysical exhaustion on the side of the psychotherapist (Marks-Tarlow, 2021).

Meanwhile, to our knowledge, no direct research on neuronal or psychophysiological synchronization between a specialist and a patient in online psychological support has been conducted so far. A few years ago, Koole and Tschacher (Koole and Tschacher, 2016) indicated that future research should establish whether there are significant differences in interpersonal synchronization between live and virtual contacts.

Brain and online environment

Selected fragments of knowledge and hypotheses on the neurobiological correlates of bonding in interpersonal relationships, including professional psychological help, have been described in the above subsections. However, can this knowledge be directly translated into the creation of a distance bond, called e-attachment in this book?

According to our knowledge, there have been no direct studies examining the brain's correlates of attachment that is created remotely through the Internet and remote communication devices. At the same time, it should be noted that many studies on neuroimaging use a methodology based on the exposure of images to the screen and the examination of the brain or physiological response to them. Therefore there is a chance to, at least, assume approximately what biological structures and physiological processes may be associated with interpersonal relationships on the "screen". In addition, there are other studies that take into account devices, social networks or other contemporary elements of culture that enable the maintenance of various interpersonal relationships, and in the context of this chapter will help to indirectly presume about the nature of these phenomena.

Social networks and the brain on the Internet

It seems that while there may be some differences, it is likely that our brains process relationships, especially in terms of social networks in real and live, in a fairly similar way. This is indicated by the issues of cognitive abilities that must be involved in such relationship processing (Dunbar, 2015; Dunbar et al., 2015). Today, a number of social interactions have moved onto the Internet and take place through websites, especially social networks and communication devices. It also makes it possible to study these interactions on both sides, meaning that through online activity we can also learn something about human interactions in reality. The Internet gives the opportunity to systematically study social and interpersonal phenomena in relation to such indicators as the number of friends on social networks, the level of activity on online forums, subscriptions, tagging, likes, etc.

This can be confirmed by one of the studies by Kanai et al., (2012) investigating the number of people in social networks – real and online (e.g. the number of people's friends on Facebook), comparing MRI scans of the respondents. It turned out that variation in the number of friends on Facebook strongly and significantly predicted gray matter volume in left middle temporal gyrus, right posterior superior temporal sulcus and right entorhinal cortex. In addition, the gray matter density of the amygdala, which was previously related to the size of real-world social networks, was also correlated to the size of the online social network.

The differences may be manifested in the fact that for online social networks, the gray matter volume is slightly greater in the posterior areas of the middle temporal gyrus, the superior temporal furrow and the right entorhinal cortex, while the right amygdala is related to the size of the social network in the real world. This is probably related to the need for high associative memory skills, which is necessary to maintain many online friendships, which is not so much needed in real-world relationships (fewer friends, and these friends are better known, do not require special diagnosis) (Kanai et al., 2012). Research on associative memory in the field of name matching has just shown an association with the right entorhinal cortex (R. Sperling et al., 2003; R. A. Sperling et al., 2001).

At the same time, it should be added that the research did not find associations with the size of online social networks in the cortical frontal parietal circuit connected so far with a network of mirror neurons and associated with the function of understanding the actions and intentions of other people, and no correlation with the medial prefrontal cortex and temporoparietal junction or with regions involved in mentalizing and adopting the perspective of others (Firth et al., 2019). Although there are obvious differences between functioning in social networks and building close relationships, including a therapeutic relationship, in the absence of other research reports, it is tempting to ask: of the above studies, the relationship on the Internet will be significantly different from the relationship in fact with a lower level of understanding the intentions of others and mentalization? A similar question has already been asked in the literature, and it relates directly to the creation of a therapeutic relationship (Siegel et al., 2021; Weinberg and Rolnick, 2019).

It should also be mentioned that research shows that the majority of the Internet users of social networking sites on the Internet supplement their existing prior social relationships in fact, maintaining, enhancing or otherwise perpetuating existing relationships in the real world. Many specialists also emphasize that in professional psychological assistance the combined model (live meetings supplemented with remote meetings) is the most optimal (Hughez, 2021; Weinberg and Rolnick, 2019).

Moving in and out on the internet

We can also look at online relations as the world of rewards and punishments, reinforcements and extinction, acceptance or rejection. However, in the real world, acceptance and rejection can be very discreet, ambiguous and susceptible to the interpretation of the recipient, while on the Internet, especially in social media, they are often clearer and even countable – through the number of likes, followers or direct hate (Firth et al., 2019). This immediate, unambiguous feedback must have a large impact on the participants of the interaction, for example it can be addictive, define, strengthen or lower self-esteem, become addictive, cause the desire to please others or the desire to provoke others. Research shows that emotions, self-esteem and self-image – especially of young internet users, can also be modulated by cyberbullying or exclusion from groups within websites, ultimately resulting in a feeling of loneliness and related feelings of depression and anxiety, and even the risk of suicide (Daly, 2018; Hamm et al., 2015; Lin et al., 2016; Twenge et al., 2017; Vannucci et al., 2017).

Some studies using functional fMRI indicated that social rejection would activate some of the same brain regions as physical pain sensation, mainly increased activity of dorsal anterior cingulate cortex, insula and the right ventral prefrontal cortex (Eisenberger, 2012; Eisenberger et al., 2003). Subsequent meta-analyzes on this topic showed increased activation of such brain regions as left inferior orbito-frontal cortex, right anterior insula, right anterior cingulate cortex, the left inferior orbito-frontal cortex and the right caudate nucleus, which, according to the authors of these meta-analyzes, is in contradiction with previous studies and testifies to a slightly different that physical pain experienced in rejection (Cacioppo et al., 2013). The authors hypothesize that these areas may reflect social insecurity, rumination, anxiety and social needs. It should be added that the above research was conducted not in a real situation, in a holistic social context, but with the use of a known Cyberball procedure (computer program), which may suggest issues related to the activation of brain areas in virtual situations.

Other studies by Puetz et al., (2014) used fMRI and the Cyberball procedure to study children's social rejection and exclusion. The subjects were children who experienced early separation from the object of attachment and were adopted, that is experiencing early life stress, and the control group, children without early stress. During the experimentally generated situation of social exclusion (Cyberball), children with early life stress, compared to the control group, showed reduced activation in the dorsal anterior cingulate cortex and the dorsolateral prefrontal cortex and reduced connectivity between dorsal anterior cingulate cortex and dorsolateral prefrontal cortex, areas believed to be involved in affect regulation. In addition, children in the study group also showed increased neuronal activation in areas of the brain involved in memory, arousal and threat-related processing (median temporal gyrus, thalamus, ventral tegmental area).

The above results, although inconsistent, may indicate that rejection, both in the real and the virtual world, will be reflected in neural circuits similar to those of physical pain or other types of discomfort (psychological/social pain?). In addition, early-life survivors of attachment trauma will also experience rejection neural differently than non-traumatized individuals in an experimental computer-based procedure, possibly showing less affect regulation and other important cognitive functions. Other studies have also shown that internet rejection increases the activity of brain areas strongly related to social cognition and real-world rejection (medial prefrontal cortex) in both children and adults (Achterberg et al., 2017; Crone and Konijn, 2018; Grossmann, 2013).

A very important though simplified reward system is the use of emoticons and other graphic symbols. An example is the popular "Like" icon. The studies by Bakshi et al., (Bakhshi et al., 2014) found that participants were much more likely to like photos containing human faces than Instagram items; however, later research also showed the opposite (Sherman et al., 2018). The results also showed that getting a lot of likes on content on social networking sites such as Instagram causes activation of the nucleus accumbens and the ventromedial prefrontal cortex (Sherman et al., 2016) and the experience of sharing information with others elicits a response in the ventral tegmental area (Tamir and Mitchell, 2012). The above-mentioned structures identified with the reward system, and what is more – the activation of these circuits resulted in increased attention (Achterberg et al., 2017; Sherman et al., 2016). Likewise, liking triggered similar areas of the brain that can be broken down into several categories:

- regions associated with reward processing and prosocial behavior, including the ventral striatum and ventromedial prefrontal cortex,
- with greater activation of the dorsal striatum, including the caudate nucleus, shell and eyeball – structures that are probably important in decision-making,
- midbrain and amygdala – that is, related to reward processing in various contexts,
- upper lateral occipital cortex, fusiform gyrus, temporal-parietal connections – associated with facial recognition and mentalization.

Thus, along with receiving and giving likes, very broad structures of the brain are activated, including those responsible for experiencing reward and prosocial behavior, and the activation of these structures is on the one hand more or less similar to those that are activated in the real world, and at the same time are extended to the above-mentioned brain structures. It can be presumed that in this case, a kind of self-reinforcing feedback loop is created in the virtual world, where both getting and giving likes can be a strong pursuit of online bonds.

Is the internet more exciting than relationships?

From an evolutionary and temperamental point of view, information-seeking is one of those properties that, on an individual and group level, increases the chances of survival and gives the possibility of appropriate neurophysiological and developmental stimulation. In this respect, the Internet will be a strong medium providing very strong incentives and rewards. The search process on the Internet may involve the "seeking" circuits described by Jaak Panksepp, which reflect an evolutionary mechanism to search for information in the environment that gives survival, from such primary as the location of food or a loved one who will help in protection, to important in today's social world, things like a link to a social networking site, forum or knowledge about others. The seeker system is stimulated by dopamine projected from the ventral tegmental area, dopamine is released each time it searches its environment, including the Internet. This puts the body in a state of well-being, sometimes even euphoria, and creates a feedback loop in which further exploration is strengthened (Parsons, 2017).

Going further, one can say, following Wegner and Ward, (2013), that the Internet is more than an information store and an external type of memory in which we can effectively search for information. The Internet began to perform the functions that relatives and friends had so far performed, that is, before the era of the Internet, when we wanted to obtain unknown information, for example about a good doctor, how to dress or where a good restaurant is located – we turned to our relatives and to a network of friends. Currently, we first turn to the Internet for this knowledge. In the context of the theory of ties, the Internet has a certain advantage over loved ones – it is available everywhere and at any time – much more than a partner or attachment figure, jokingly speaking – the Internet does not go anywhere. Second, the Internet in ordinary life situations usually has much more and more knowledge than any close person in the environment, and the data on the Internet is constantly updated. This can have both good and negative consequences. On the one hand, relatives no longer have to be burdened with one of the types of support – in informational support and storing a large amount of information, they no longer have to hold a large amount of information, because others do not expect it anymore. This may be reflected in creativity and the use of creative problem solving (part of the memory store and attention is released). On the other hand, attachment motivation is transferred from real social relations to the Internet, creating the basis for the impoverishment of real interpersonal relations and behavioral addictions. To what extent will people be willing to seek professional help from a psychologist and other mental health specialists, in the context of the fact that the Internet offers a whole range of information, diagnosis and self-treatment tips? One more aspect – on the cognitive level, people can release their biological memory banks onto digital banks, which may be reflected in their motivation to stimulate memory, memories, and information processing abilities. On the cognitive level, users may begin to replace their biological memory banks with digital storage. A further consequence may be an interference with the user's motivation and ability to process information and form new memories.

Future directions

The chapter dealt with the hypothetical interdependencies between building interpersonal relations and the bond in remote communication, devices and the Internet, and the neuronal and physiological correlates of these relations. It is important to emphasize the word "hypothetical" because at the moment there is not enough data from research on such phenomena. In many places in this text, we referred to research from synonymous areas in order to be able to assume and speculate on whether the relationship between a specialist and a patient in online contact will be the same. The research to date is inconclusive, some of them show a surprising similarity between the neural correlates of live and online contact, while others give grounds to think of them as different and non-comparable phenomena. However, one should also be aware of a methodological paradox, consisting in the fact that a lot of research on the brain is carried out during typical laboratory experiments, where stimuli (including social stimuli) are given to the test subjects on the monitor screen – so they are basically deprived of the overall ecological and social context.

There is no doubt that further research in this area will be not only very interesting but also very necessary in the context of the irreversible process of using modern technologies in the work of a psychologist and psychotherapist. Detailed knowledge (also neurobiological) about the similarity of building interpersonal bonds, including in the relationship between the psychologist and the patient in a direct and online situation, is needed. Similarities and differences may indicate the need to modify diagnostic and therapeutic procedures, including the use of new technologies, for example virtual reality. On the basis of such research, it will also be possible to conclude about the effectiveness of online psychological help.

References

Achterberg, M., van Duijvenvoorde, A.C.K., van der Meulen, M., Euser, S., Bakermans-Kranenburg, M.J., Crone, E.A. (2017). The neural and behavioral correlates of social evaluation in childhood. *Developmental Cognitive Neuroscience*, 24, 107–117. 10.1016/J.DCN.2017.02.007

Ahnert, L., Gunnar, M.R., Lamb, M.E., Barthel, M. (2004). Transition to child care: Associations with infant-mother attachment, infant negative emotion, and cortisol elevations. *Child Development*, 75(3), 639–650. 10.1111/j.1467-8624.2004.00698.x

Bakhshi, S., Shamma, D.A., Gilbert, E. (2014). Faces engage us: Photos with faces attract more likes and comments on instagram. *Conference on Human Factors in Computing Systems – Proceedings*, 965–974. 10.1145/2556288.2557403

Beintner, I., Görlich, D., Berger, T., Ebert, D.D., Zeiler, M., Herrero Camarano, R., Waldherr, K., Jacobi, C. (2019). Interrelations between participant and intervention characteristics, process variables and outcomes in online interventions: A protocol for overarching analyses within and across seven clinical trials in ICare. *Internet Interventions*, 16, 86–97. 10.1016/J.INVENT.2018.05.001

Benuzzi, F., Pugnaghi, M., Meletti, S., Lui, F., Serafini, M., Baraldi, P., Nichelli, P. (2007). Processing the socially relevant parts of faces. *Brain Research Bulletin*, 74(5). 10.1016/j.brainresbull.2007.07.010

Bernard, K., Dozier, M. (2010). Examining infants' cortisol responses to laboratory tasks among children varying in attachment disorganization: Stress reactivity or return to baseline? *Developmental Psychology*, 46(6). 10.1037/a0020660

Bowlby, J. (1969). *Attachment and Loss* (2nd eds.). Basic Books. http://www.amazon.com/Attachment-Volume-Basic-Books-Classics/dp/0465005438

Bowlby, J. (1982). Attachment and Loss. Volume I Attachment. In *Basic Books*: Vol. I.

Bretherton, I., Munholland, K.A. (2016). The Internal Working Model Construct in Light of Contemporary Neuroimaging Research. *Handbook of Attachment: Theory, Research, and Clinical Applications*, 4, 63–88.

Buchheim, A., Erk, S., George, C., Kächele, H., Kircher, T., Martius, P., Pokorny, D., Ruchsow, M., Spitzer, M., Walter, H. (2008). Neural correlates of attachment trauma in borderline personality disorder: A functional magnetic resonance imaging study. *Psychiatry Research: Neuroimaging*, 163(3), 223–235. 10.1016/J.PSCYCHRESNS.2007.07.001

Buchheim, A., Erk, S., George, C., Kächele, H., Ruchsow, M., Spitzer, M., Kircher, T., Walter, H. (2006). Measuring Attachment Representation in an fMRI Environment: A Pilot Study. *Psychopathology*, 39(3), 144–152. 10.1159/000091800

Buss, D.M. (2019). Evolutionary psychology: The new science of the mind. In *Evolutionary Psychology: The New Science of the Mind*. Taylor and Francis. 10.4324/9780429061417/EVOLUTIONARY-PSYCHOLOGY-DAVID-BUSS

Cacioppo, S., Frum, C., Asp, E., Weiss, R.M., Lewis, J.W., Cacioppo, J.T. (2013). A quantitative meta-analysis of functional imaging studies of social rejection. *Scientific Reports*, 3. 10.1038/srep02027

Callaghan, B.L., Tottenham, N. (2016). The neuro-environmental loop of plasticity: A cross-species analysis of parental effects on emotion circuitry development following typical and adverse caregiving. In *Neuropsychopharmacology*, 41(1). 10.1038/npp.2015.204

Carter, S.C. (2014). Oxytocin pathways and the evolution of human behavior. In *Annual Review of Psychology*, 65, (pp. 17–39). 10.1146/annurev-psych-010213-115110

Carter, S.C., Devries-Courtney, A., Lowell, G. (1995). Physiological substrates of mammalian monogamy: The prairie vole model. *Neuroscience and Biobehavioral Reviews*, 19(2), 303–314. 10.1016/0149-7634(94)00070-H

Chambers, J. (2017). The Neurobiology of Attachment: From Infancy to Clinical Outcomes, 45(4), 542–563. 10.1521/PDPS.2017.45.4.542

Chaminade, T., Hodgins, J., Kawato, M. (2007). Anthropomorphism influences perception of computer-animated characters' actions. *Social Cognitive and Affective Neuroscience*, 2(3), 206–216. 10.1093/SCAN/NSM017

Coan, J. (2019). Toward a Neuroscience of Attachment. In J. Cassidy & P. R. Shaver (Eds.), *Handbook of Attachment* (Third edit). Guilford Press.

Coan, J.A., Schaefer, H.S., Davidson, R.J. (2006). Lending a hand: Social regulation of the neural response to threat. *Psychological Science*, 17(12). 10.1111/j.1467-9280.2006.01832.x

Conner, O.L., Siegle, G.J., McFarland, A.M., Silk, J.S., Ladouceur, C.D., Dahl, R.E., Coan, J.A., Ryan, N.D., Laks, J. (2012). Mom-it helps when you're right here! Attenuation of neural stress markers in anxious youths whose caregivers are present during fMRI. *PloS One*, 7(12). 10.1371/JOURNAL.PONE.0050680

Cozolino, L. (2014). *The Neuroscience of Human Relationships: Attachment and the Developing Social Brain* (2nd eds.). W. W. Norton & Company.

Crone, E.A., & Konijn, E.A. (2018). Media use and brain development during adolescence. *Nature Communications*, 9(1), 1–10. 10.1038/s41467-018-03126-x

Daly, M. (2018). Social-Media Use May Explain Little of the Recent Rise in Depressive Symptoms Among Adolescent Girls. *Clinical Psychological Science*, 6(3), 295. 10.1177/21 67702617750869

Dunbar, R.I.M. (2015). Do online social media cut through the constraints that limit the size of offline social networks? *Royal Society Open Science*, 3(1). 10.1098/RSOS.150292

Dunbar, R.I.M., Arnaboldi, V., Conti, M., Passarella, A. (2015). The structure of online social networks mirrors those in the offline world. *Social Networks*, 43. 10.1016/j.socnet.2 015.04.005

Eisenberger, N.I. (2012). The neural bases of social pain: Evidence for shared representations with physical pain. *Psychosomatic Medicine*, 74(2), 126–135. 10.1097/PSY.0b013e31 82464dd1

Eisenberger, N.I., Lieberman, M.D., Williams, K.D. (2003). Does rejection hurt? An FMRI study of social exclusion. *Science (New York, N.Y.)*, 302(5643), 290–292. 10.1126/ SCIENCE.1089134

Firth, J., Torous, J., Stubbs, B., Firth, J.A., Steiner, G.Z., Smith, L., Alvarez-Jimenez, M., Gleeson, J., Vancampfort, D., Armitage, C.J., Sarris, J. (2019). The "online brain": how the Internet may be changing our cognition. *World Psychiatry*, 18(2), 119–129. 10.1002/ WPS.20617

Frith, U., Frith, C.D. (2003). Development and neurophysiology of mentalizing. *Philosophical Transactions of the Royal Society B: Biological Sciences*, 358(1431), 459. 10. 1098/RSTB.2002.1218

Gray, S.A.O., Lipschutz, R.S., Scheeringa, M.S. (2018). Young Children's Physiological Reactivity During Memory Recall: Associations with Posttraumatic Stress and Parent Physiological Synchrony. *Journal of Abnormal Child Psychology*, 46(4), 871. 10.1007/S1 0802-017-0326-1

Grossmann, T. (2013). The role of medial prefrontal cortex in early social cognition. In *Frontiers in Human Neuroscience*. 10.3389/fnhum.2013.00340

Hamann, S.B., Ely, T.D., Grafton, S.T., Kilts, C.D. (1999). Amygdala activity related to enhanced memory for pleasant and aversive stimuli. *Nature Neuroscience*, 2(3). 10.1038/ 6404

Hamm, M.P., Newton, A.S., Chisholm, A., Shulhan, J., Milne, A., Sundar, P., Ennis, H., Scott, S.D., Hartling, L. (2015). Prevalence and Effect of Cyberbullying on Children and Young People: A Scoping Review of Social Media Studies. *JAMA Pediatrics*, 169(8), 770–777. 10.1001/JAMAPEDIATRICS.2015.0944

Hansen, S., Harthon, C., Wallin, E., Löfberg, L., Svensson, K. (1991). The effects of 6-OHDA-induced dopamine depletions in the ventral or dorsal striatum on maternal and sexual behavior in the female rat. *Pharmacology, Biochemistry, and Behavior*, 39(1), 71–77. 10.1016/0091-3057(91)90399-M

Healey, D.M., Gopin, C.B., Grossman, B.R., Campbell, S.B., Halperin, J.M. (2010). Mother-child dyadic synchrony is associated with better functioning in hyperactive/ inattentive preschool children. *Journal of Child Psychology and Psychiatry, and Allied Disciplines*, 51(9), 1058–1066. 10.1111/J.1469-7610.2010.02220.X

Hertsgaard, L., Gunnar, M., Erickson, M.F., Nachmias, M. (1995). Adrenocortical Responses to the Strange Situation in Infants with Disorganized/Disoriented Attachment Relationships. *Child Development*, 66(4). 10.1111/j.1467-8624.1995.tb00925.x

Hofer, M.A. (2006). Psychobiological roots of early attachment. *Current Directions in Psychological Science*, 15(2). 10.1111/j.0963-7214.2006.00412.x

Howell, B.R., Grand, A.P., Mccormack, K.M., Shi, Y., Laprarie, J.L., Maestripieri, D., Styner, M.A., Sanchez, M.M. (2014). Early adverse experience increases emotional re-activity in juvenile rhesus macaques: Relation to amygdala volume. In *Developmental Psychobiology*,56(8). 10.1002/dev.21237

Hughez, D. (2021). Synchronizing Neurological States of Emotion in Family Therapy While Online. In D. J. Siegel, A. Schore, L. Cozolino (Eds.), *Interpersonal Neurobiology and Clinical Practice* (1th eds.), p. 368. W. W. Norton & Company.

Humphreys, K.L., Zeanah, C.H. (2015). Deviations from the Expectable Environment in Early Childhood and Emerging Psychopathology. In *Neuropsychopharmacology*, 40(1). 10.1038/npp.2014.165

Iacoboni, M. (2008). *Mirroring People: the Science of Empathy and How We Connect with Others* (1th eds.), p. 316). Farrar, Straus and Giroux. https://books.google.com/books/about/ Mirroring_People.html?hl=pl&id=FEWWzxLlP8YC

Iacoboni, M. (2009a). Imitation, empathy, and mirror neurons. In *Annual Review of Psychology*, 60. 10.1146/annurev.psych.60.110707.163604

Iacoboni, M. (2009b). Neurobiology of imitation. In *Current Opinion in Neurobiology*, 19(6). 10.1016/j.conb.2009.09.008

Insel, T.R., Fernald, R.D. (2004). How the brain processes social information: Searching for the social brain. In *Annual Review of Neuroscience* (27). 10.1146/annurev.neuro.2 7.070203.144148

Jasper, K., Weise, C., Conrad, I., Andersson, G., Hiller, W., Kleinstäuber, M. (2014). The working alliance in a randomized controlled trial comparing Internet-based self-help and face-to-face cognitive behavior therapy for chronic tinnitus. *Internet Interventions*, 1(2), 49–57. 10.1016/J.INVENT.2014.04.002

Jiang, J., Dai, B., Peng, D., Zhu, C., Liu, L., Lu, C. (2012). Neural Synchronization during Face-to-Face Communication. *Journal of Neuroscience*, 32(45), 16064–16069. 10.1523/ JNEUROSCI.2926-12.2012

Johansen, J.P., Cain, C.K., Ostroff, L.E., Ledoux, J.E. (2011). Molecular mechanisms of fear learning and memory. In *Cell*, 147(3). 10.1016/j.cell.2011.10.009

Kanai, R., Bahrami, B., Roylance, R., Rees, G. (2012). Online social network size is reflected in human brain structure. *Proceedings of the Royal Society B: Biological Sciences*, 279(1732), 1327–1334. 10.1098/RSPB.2011.1959

Kim, S., Kochanska, G. (2015). Mothers' Power Assertion, Children's Negative, Adversarial Orientation, and Future Behavior Problems in Low-Income Families: Early Maternal Responsiveness as a Moderator of the Developmental Cascade. *Journal of Family*

Psychology: JFP: Journal of the Division of Family Psychology of the American Psychological Association (Division 43), 29(1). 10.1037/A0038430

Kleinbub, J.R., Talia, A., Palmieri, A. (2020). Physiological synchronization in the clinical process: A research primer. *Journal of Counseling Psychology*, 67(4), 420–437. 10.1037/COU0000383

Koole, S.L., Tschacher, W. (2016). Synchrony in Psychotherapy: A Review and an Integrative Framework for the Therapeutic Alliance. *Frontiers in Psychology*, 7. 10.3389/FPSYG.2016.00862

Kovács, Á.M., Kühn, S., Gergely, G., Csibra, G., Brass, M. (2014). Are all beliefs equal? Implicit belief attributions recruiting core brain regions of theory of mind. *PLoS ONE*, 9(9). 10.1371/journal.pone.0106558

Lammel, S., Lim, B.K., Malenka, R.C. (2014). Reward and aversion in a heterogeneous midbrain dopamine system. *Neuropharmacology*, 76, 351–359. 10.1016/J.NEUROPHARM. 2013.03.019

Li, Z., Sturge-Apple, M.L., Liu, S., Davies, P.T. (2020). Parent-adolescent physiological synchrony: Moderating effects of adolescent emotional insecurity. *Psychophysiology*, 57(9), 13596. 10.1111/PSYP.13596

Lim, M.M., Young, L.J. (2006). Neuropeptidergic regulation of affiliative behavior and social bonding in animals. *Hormones and Behavior*, 50(4), 506–517. 10.1016/J.YHBEH.2 006.06.028

Lin, L.Y., Sidani, J.E., Shensa, A., Radovic, A., Miller, E., Colditz, J.B., Hoffman, B.L., Giles, L.M., Primack, B.A. (2016). Association between social media use and depression among U.S. young adults. *Depression and Anxiety*, 33(4), 323–331. 10.1002/DA.22466

Luijk, M.P.C.M., Saridjan, N., Tharner, A., van Ijzendoorn, M.H., Bakermans-Kranenburg, M.J., Jaddoe, V.W.V., Hofman, A., Verhulst, F.C., Tiemeier, H. (2010). Attachment, depression, and cortisol: Deviant patterns in insecure-resistant and disorganized infants. *Developmental Psychobiology*, 52(5). 10.1002/dev.20446

Lungwitz, E.A., Stuber, G.D., Johnson, P.L., Dietrich, A.D., Schartz, N., Hanrahan, B., Shekhar, A., Truitt, W.A. (2014). The role of the medial prefrontal cortex in regulating social familiarity-induced anxiolysis. *Neuropsychopharmacology*, 39(4), 1009–1019. 10.103 8/npp.2013.302

Lupien, S.J., Parent, S., Evans, A.C., Tremblay, R.E., Zelazo, P.D., Corbo, V., Pruessner, J.C., Séguin, J.R. (2011). Larger amygdala but no change in hippocampal volume in q10-year-old children exposed to maternal depressive symptomatology since birth. *Proceedings of the National Academy of Sciences of the United States of America*, 108(34). 10.1073/pnas.1105371108

Lyons-Ruth, K., Pechtel, P., Yoon, S.A., Anderson, C.M., Teicher, M.H. (2016). Disorganized attachment in infancy predicts greater amygdala volume in adulthood. *Behavioural Brain Research*, 308, 83–93. 10.1016/j.bbr.2016.03.050

Marci, C.D., Ham, J., Moran, E., Orr, S.P. (2007). Physiologic correlates of perceived therapist empathy and social-emotional process during psychotherapy. *The Journal of Nervous and Mental Disease*, 195(2), 103–111. 10.1097/01.NMD.0000253731.71025.FC

Marks-Tarlow, T. (2021). Birds of Feather. The Importance of Interpersonal Synchrony in Psychotherapy. In D. J. Siegel, A. Schore, & L. Cozolino (Eds.), *Interpersonal Neurobiology and Clinical Practice* (1th ed., p. 368). W. W. Norton & Company.

Marmarosh, C.L., Markin, R.D., & Spiegel, E.B. (2013). Attachment in group psychotherapy. In *Attachment in Group Psychotherapy*. American Psychological Association. 10.1037/14186-000

Mehta, M.A., Golembo, N.I., Nosarti, C., Colvert, E., Mota, A., Williams, S.C.R., Rutter, M., Sonuga-Barke, E.J.S. (2009). Amygdala, hippocampal and corpus callosum size following severe early institutional deprivation: the English and Romanian Adoptees study pilot. *Journal of Child Psychology and Psychiatry, and Allied Disciplines*, 50(8). 10.1111/j.1469-7610.2009.02084.x

Morrone-Strupinsky, J.V., Depue, R.A. (2005). A neurobehavioral model of affiliative bonding: Implications for conceptualizing a human trait of affiliation. *Behavioral and Brain Sciences*, 28(3).

Moutsiana, C., Johnstone, T., Murray, L., Fearon, P., Cooper, P.J., Pliatsikas, C., Goodyer, I., Halligan, S.L. (2015). Insecure attachment during infancy predicts greater amygdala volumes in early adulthood. *Journal of Child Psychology and Psychiatry and Allied Disciplines*, 56(5), 540–548. 10.1111/jcpp.12317

Norcross, J.C., Lambert, M.J. (2018). Psychotherapy Relationships That Work III. *Psychotherapy*, 55(4). 10.1037/pst0000193

Ochsner, K.N., Silvers, J.A., Buhle, J.T. (2012). Functional imaging studies of emotion regulation: a synthetic review and evolving model of the cognitive control of emotion. *Annals of the New York Academy of Sciences*, 1251, 1–24. 10.1111/J.1749-6632.2012. 06751.X

Parsons, T.D. (2017). Cyberpsychology and the Brain. In *Cyberpsychology and the Brain*. 10.1 017/9781316151204

Pelphrey, K.A., Carter, E.J. (2008). Brain mechanisms for social perception: lessons from autism and typical development. *Annals of the New York Academy of Sciences*, 1145, 283–299. 10.1196/ANNALS.1416.007

Piasecka, B., Bryniarska, A., Mróz, S., Wojszel, B., Janczura, M., Józefik, B., Siwiec-Bek, A., Taurogiński, B. (2021). From march 2020 to march 2021 – psychotherapists about working in the covid-19 pandemic. Collective Autoethnography. *Psychotherapy*, 2(197), 9–27. 10.12740/PT/139681

Pihlaja, S., Stenberg, J.H., Joutsenniemi, K., Mehik, H., Ritola, V., Joffe, G. (2018). Therapeutic alliance in guided internet therapy programs for depression and anxiety disorders – A systematic review. *Internet Interventions*, 11, 1–10. 10.1016/J.INVENT.201 7.11.005

Puetz, V.B., Kohn, N., Dahmen, B., Zvyagintsev, M., Schüppen, A., Schultz, R.T., Heim, C.M., Fink, G.R., Herpertz-Dahlmann, B., Konrad, K. (2014). Neural response to social rejection in children with early separation experiences. *Journal of the American Academy of Child and Adolescent Psychiatry*, 53(12), 1328–1337. 10.1016/J.JAAC.2014.09.004

Reilly, E.B., Gunnar, M.R. (2019). Neglect, HPA axis reactivity, and development. In *International Journal of Developmental Neuroscience*, 78. 10.1016/j.ijdevneu.2019.07.010

Rizzolatti, G., Fadiga, L., Gallese, V., Fogassi, L. (1996). Premotor cortex and the recognition of motor actions. *Cognitive Brain Research*, 3(2), 131–141. 10.1016/0926-641 0(95)00038-0

Rolls, E.T. (2007). Emotion elicited by primary reinforcers and following stimulus-reinforcement association learning. In J. Coan, J. Allen (Eds.), *Handbook of Emotion Elicitation and Assessment*. (pp. 137–157). Oxford University Press.

Saxe, R., Kanwisher, N. (2003). People thinking about thinking people: The role of the temporo-parietal junction in "theory of mind". *NeuroImage*, 19(4). 10.1016/S1053-811 9(03)00230-1

Schalinski, I., Teicher, M.H., Rockstroh, B. (2019). Early neglect is a key determinant of adult hair cortisol concentration and is associated with increased vulnerability to trauma in a transdiagnostic sample. *Psychoneuroendocrinology*, 108, 35–42. 10.1016/J.PSYNEUEN.2019. 06.007

Schore, A. (2003). *Affect Dysregulation and the Repair of the Self*. In New York & London: WW Norton.

Schore, A. (2009). Relational trauma and the developing right brain: An interface of psychoanalytic self psychology and neuroscience. *Annals of the New York Academy of Sciences*, 1159, 189–203. 10.1111/j.1749-6632.2009.04474.x

Schore, A.N. (2014). The right brain is dominant in psychotherapy. *Psychotherapy (Chicago, Ill.)*, 51(3), 388–397. 10.1037/A0037083

Schore, A.N. (2021). The Interpersonal Neurobiology of Intersubjectivity. *Frontiers in Psychology*, 12, 1366. 10.3389/FPSYG.2021.648616/BIBTEX

Seay, B., Harlow, H.F. (1965). Maternal separation in the rhesus monkey. *Journal of Nervous and Mental Disease*, 140(6). 10.1097/00005053-196506000-00006

Shahrokh, D.K., Zhang, T.Y., Diorio, J., Gratton, A., Meaney, M.J. (2010). Oxytocin-dopamine interactions mediate variations in maternal behavior in the rat. *Endocrinology*, 151(5), 2276–2286. 10.1210/EN.2009-1271

Sheridan, M.A., McLaughlin, K.A. (2014). Dimensions of early experience and neural development: Deprivation and threat. In *Trends in Cognitive Sciences*, 18(11). 10.1016/ j.tics.2014.09.001

Sherman, L.E., Hernandez, L.M., Greenfield, P.M., Dapretto, M. (2018). What the brain 'Likes': neural correlates of providing feedback on social media. *Social Cognitive and Affective Neuroscience*, 13(7), 699–707. 10.1093/SCAN/NSY051

Sherman, L.E., Payton, A.A., Hernandez, L.M., Greenfield, P.M., Dapretto, M. (2016). The Power of the Like in Adolescence: Effects of Peer Influence on Neural and Behavioral Responses to Social Media. *Psychological Science*, 27(7), 1027–1035. 10.1177/ 0956797616645673

Siegel, D.J. (2007). *Reflections on The Mindful Brain*. The Mindful Brain: Reflection and Attunement in the Cultivation of Well-Being.

Siegel, D.J. (2015). Interpersonal Neurobiology as a Lens into the Development of Wellbeing and Reslience. *Children Australia*, 40(2), 160–164. 10.1017/CHA.2015.7

Siegel, D.J., Schore, A., Cozolino, L. (2021). *Interpersonal Neurobiology and Clinical Practice* (1th ed., p. 368). W. W. Norton & Company.

Spangler, G., Grossmann, K.E. (1993). Biobehavioral Organization in Securely and Insecurely Attached Infants. *Child Development*, 64(5). 10.1111/j.1467-8624.1993.tb02 962.x

Spangler, G., Schieche, M. (1998). Emotional and Adrenocortical Responses of Infants to the Strange Situation: The Differential Function of Emotional Expression. *International Journal of Behavioral Development*, 22(4). 10.1080/016502598384126

Sperling, R.A., Bates, J.F., Cocchiarella, A.J., Schacter, D.L., Rosen, B.R., Albert, M.S. (2001). Encoding novel face-name associations: a functional MRI study. *Human Brain Mapping*, 14(3), 129–139. 10.1002/HBM.1047

Sperling, R., Chua, E., Cocchiarella, A., Rand-Giovannetti, E., Poldrack, R., Schacter, D.L., Albert, M. (2003). Putting names to faces: Successful encoding of associative memories activates the anterior hippocampal formation. *NeuroImage*, 20(2). 10.1016/S1 053-8119(03)00391-4

Sucala, M., Schnur, J.B., Constantino, M.J., Miller, S.J., Brackman, E.H., Montgomery, G.H. (2012). The Therapeutic Relationship in E-Therapy for Mental Health: A Systematic Review. *Journal of Medical Internet Research*, 14(4), 110 https://Www.Jmir. Org/2012/4/E110, 14(4), e2084. 10.2196/JMIR.2084

Tamir, D.I., Mitchell, J.P. (2012). Disclosing information about the self is intrinsically rewarding. *Proceedings of the National Academy of Sciences of the United States of America*, 109(21), 8038–8043. 10.1073/PNAS.1202129109/SUPPL_FILE/PNAS. 201202129SI.PDF

Teicher, M.H., Samson, J.A., Anderson, C.M., Ohashi, K. (2016). The effects of childhood maltreatment on brain structure, function and connectivity. In *Nature Reviews Neuroscience*, 17(10). 10.1038/nrn.2016.111

Tourunen, A., Kykyri, V.L., Seikkula, J., Kaartinen, J., Tolvanen, A., Penttonen, M. (2020). Sympathetic nervous system synchrony: An exploratory study of its relationship with the therapeutic alliance and outcome in couple therapy. *Psychotherapy (Chicago, Ill.)*, 57(2), 160–173. 10.1037/PST0000198

Twenge, J.M., Joiner, T.E., Rogers, M.L., Martin, G.N. (2017). Increases in Depressive Symptoms, Suicide-Related Outcomes, and Suicide Rates Among U.S. Adolescents After 2010 and Links to Increased New Media Screen Time: *Clinical Psychological Science*, 6(1), 3–17. 10.1177/2167702617723376

Vannucci, A., Flannery, K.M., Ohannessian, C.M.C. (2017). Social media use and anxiety in emerging adults. *Journal of Affective Disorders*, 207. 10.1016/j.jad.2016.08.040

Varker, T., Brand, R.M., Ward, J., Terhaag, S., Phelps, A. (2018). Efficacy of Synchronous Telepsychology Interventions for People With Anxiety, Depression, Posttraumatic Stress Disorder, and Adjustment Disorder: A Rapid Evidence Assessment. *Psychological Services*. 10.1037/ser0000239

Wallin, D. (2007). *Attachment in Psychotherapy* (1th ed.). Guilford Publications. 10.1 080/15228870802111856

Wegner, D., Ward, A. (2013). *The Internet Has Become the External Hard Drive for Our Memories*. Scientific American.

Weinberg, H., Rolnick, A. (2019). Theory and Practice of Online Therapy. In H. Weinberg & A. Rolnick (Eds.), *Theory and Practice of Online Therapy: Internet-delivered Interventions for Individuals, Groups, Families, and Organizations* (1th ed.). Routledge. 10.4324/9781315545530

White, L.O., Ising, M., von Klitzing, K., Sierau, S., Michel, A., Klein, A.M., Andreas, A., Keil, J., Quintero, L., Müller-Myhsok, B., Uhr, M., Gausche, R., Manly, J.T., Crowley, M.J., Kirschbaum, C., Stalder, T. (2017). Reduced hair cortisol after maltreatment mediates externalizing symptoms in middle childhood and adolescence. *Journal of Child Psychology and Psychiatry and Allied Disciplines*, 58(9). 10.1111/jcpp.12700

White, L.O., Schulz, C.C., Schoett, M.J.S., Kungl, M.T., Keil, J., Borelli, J.L., Vrtička, P. (2020). Conceptual Analysis: A Social Neuroscience Approach to Interpersonal Interaction in the Context of Disruption and Disorganization of Attachment (NAMDA). *Frontiers in Psychiatry*, 11, 1437. 10.3389/FPSYT.2020.517372/BIBTEX

Woody, M.L., Feurer, C., Sosoo, E.E., Hastings, P.D., Gibb, B.E. (2016). Synchrony of physiological activity during mother-child interaction: moderation by maternal history of major depressive disorder. *Journal of Child Psychology and Psychiatry, and Allied Disciplines*, 57(7), 843–850. 10.1111/JCPP.12562

Young, L.J., Wang, Z. (2004). The neurobiology of pair bonding. *Nature Neuroscience 2004 7:10*, 7(10), 1048–1054. 10.1038/nn1327

Zeifman, D., Hazan, C. (1997). A process model of adult attachment formation. In S. Duck (Ed.), *Handbook of Personal Relationships: Theory, Research and Interventions (2nd ed.).* (2nd ed., pp. 179–195). John Wiley & Sons Inc. http://search.ebscohost.com/login.aspx?direct=true&db=psyh&AN=1997-08290-007&site=ehost-live

Chapter 4

Attachment based on new technologies and mental health

Mental health and disturbed attachment – psychological perspective

Mental health is a phenomenon experienced at all ages of human life in many aspects and in a way that is difficult to define unequivocally, as suggested by mental health indicators described in contemporary medical and psychological literature (Rokita et al., 2018). In the light of psychological theories and clinical experiences of a psychologist and psychotherapist, the complexity and multiplicity of diverse: biological psychological and social factors influencing the experience of various phenomena of a person's mental life during their life are confirmed (Green et al., 2010). Taking into account the wide spectrum of biological and psychosocial risk/protective factors which may affect the development of various mental difficulties and disorders, indicated in the literature and observed in the clinical practice of psychologists and psychotherapists, it is worth emphasizing the importance of shaping the mental bond built in the course of life and related to its quality attachment patterns.

According to Green et al., (2010), who studied 5.692 people as part of the National Comorbidity Survey Replication (NCS-R), 44.6% of people with mental disorders with developmental onset and 25.9–32% with adult onset experienced dysfunctional care during childhood. The psychological perspective referring to the theories of psychoanalytical and developmental theories of bonds and mentalization indicates the need to include in the diagnosis and psychological therapy the thesis about the mutual relations between the different level of experienced bond deficits and the level of psychopathology of the personality structure. Researchers and theorists of the psychoanalytic paradigm, especially the psychology of object relations, emphasize the important role of the level of personality structure maturity in defining indicators of mental health and mental disorders (Clarkin et al., 2013; Gabbard, 2013, 2015). According to the object relationship and psychodynamic theory – there are three main levels of personality structure disorders: neurotic, borderline and psychotic (Gabbard, 2013; Clarkin et al., 2013). The level of the depth of

DOI: 10.4324/9781003221043-5

disorders of the personality structure simultaneously characterizes the level of destabilization of mental health and psychopathological symptoms.

Clarkin et al., (2013) and Gabbard (2013), defining the neurotic structure of personality, indicate that it is characterized by: the presence of personality stiffness, but the lack of identity pathology (the present consolidated, stable self, developed the ability to self-observe, self-reflection, understand the symbolic nature of thoughts, to easily relate and maintaining relationships and adequate control of impulses and drives). The transfer that develops in the relationship between diagnosis and therapy (projection of a fixed pattern of relations with a significant person in the past onto the person of a diagnostician) is characterized by subtlety and affective adequacy (no excessively negative or excessively positive intensity).

Higher borderline level compared to lower borderline level, Clarkin et al., (2013) and Gabbard (2013) describe as one that is characterized by:

• Lower severity of identity pathology (consolidated identity: correct differentiation of one's own boundaries with the boundaries of others and the outside world, correctly preserved allo and autopsychic orientation, no psychotic symptoms of production),
• Lower severity of the pathology of the relationship with the object (the person's ability to establish an emotional bond with other people, no excessive hostility and paranoid distrust in the social relationship being built),
• Lower level of disorders in moral development (retained ability to adequately experience guilt),
• A smaller role of poorly integrated aggression as a regulator of experienced emotional states (no features of diffuse hostility, impulsiveness in the emotional regulation of behavior in a situation).

The psychodynamic perspective in defining the organization of the personality structure and the genesis of personality disorders emphasize the diagnosis of the level of stability of the pattern of building emotional ties and relationships with other people as an important criterion related to the different level of destabilization of the personality structure in terms of evaluation: the stability of the self-image and the level of identity maturity, the ability to self-reflection activities and experiences of other internal states, regulation of aggression, the pursuit of goals (Verheul et al., 2008). A special place in defining the criteria describing the level of destabilization of the personality structure (and thus the level of mental health quality) is played by the criterion of assessing the pattern of building an emotional bond with other people, which is based on the early childhood attachment pattern (Green et al., 2010; Gabbard, 2013; Clarkin et al., 2013).

The studies conducted so far also lead to the conclusion that insecure attachment patterns (especially anxiety-ambivalent and disorganized attachment) have been shown to be associated with experiencing high levels of anxiety and stress, demonstrating a strategy of coping with stress (Mikulincer and Florian, 1998) and with negative affect (Mikulincer, 1998b; Myers and Wells, 2015). High levels of experienced anxiety and stress are important criteria for identifying risk factors for the development of chronic emotional crises and mental disorders. Some researchers also emphasize that insecure attachment patterns may affect developmental trajectories, increasing the risk of internalizing and externalizing disorders (Ramos et al., 2016). Studies also documented the relationship between insecure attachment patterns and the severity of somatic, psychosomatic symptoms and less-specific mental health disturbances (Taylor et al., 2000). The literature indicates the interrelationships between the patterns of insecure attachment and anxiety disorders, depression, post-traumatic stress disorder (PTSD), (Beeney et al., 2015; Boldrini et al., 2020a,b), personality disorders (Kochanska and Kim, 2012), eating disorders (Eggert et al., 2007; Bamford and Halliwell, 2009; Zachrisson and Skårderud, 2010) and psychotic disorders (Korver-Nieberg, 2014; Debbané et al., 2016; Rokita et al., 2018; Boldrini et al., 2020b; Carr et al., 2018; Chatziioannidis, 2019; Lavin et al., 2020; Llewellyn-Jones, 2019; Murphy et al., 2020; Sheinbaum et al., 2020). Mikulincer and Shaver (2010), in a review of several dozen works on the relationship between attachment and depression, indicated the relationship between the insecure (anxious–avoidant) attachment pattern and depression (Bifulco et al., 2006).

In particular, research does not exclude the hypothesis that an anxious-avoidant attachment pattern may mediate the relationship between childhood trauma (violence) and a tendency to psychosis (Sheinbaum et al., 2014; Sheinbaum, 2015; Rokita et al., 2018). The results of many conducted studies indicate an important role of the anxious attachment pattern in the prediction of disorders in social functioning and somatic symptoms in adulthood (Taylor et al., 2000; Żechowski et al., 2018). In the study by Waldinger et al., (2006) trauma in childhood and insecure attachment were independent predictors of somatization in adulthood. Similar dependency – the relationship between the insecure attachment pattern and the intensification of somatic symptoms – were also indicated in their research by Riem et al. (2012). These authors also pointed to the mediating role of alexithymia and metallization disorders between the insecure attachment pattern and somatic disorders.

A specific attachment style, even insecure, is not a disorder in itself, but it is an important risk factor that determines a developmental trajectory from childhood that much more often leads to disturbances in mental health. From a medical perspective, attachment disorders are defined as the disruption of normal social interactions in infants and young children as a result of emotional neglect. They lead to deficits in building relationships in the following years of life. In response to this fact, whole groups of disorders were defined, defined as attachment disorders, which in the latest medical classifications ICD 11 (Krawczyk and Święcicki, 2020) and DSM -5 (2013) were categorized in the group of disorders related to trauma and stress and are recognized as early PTSD variant (Table 4.1).

Table 4.1 Attachment disorders according to ICD 11 (WHO, 2019)

Reactive Attachment Disorder

Required traits:
* Episodes of inadequate care:
  * Further disregard the child's basic emotional (comfort, progress, feelings) and physical needs
  * Many new caregivers (e.g. repeated changes in foster care providers)
  * Upbringing in an unusual conditions (e.g. institutions) that preclude formation of stable selective attachments
  * Bullying
* Clearly abnormal attachment behaviors towards adult caregivers, characterized by a persistent and ubiquitous pattern of inhibition and emotional withdrawal:
  * Minimal search for comfort in restlessness
  * Infrequent or minimal response to comfort when it is offered
* Inadequate care is responsible for the persistent and the ubiquitous pattern of inhibited, emotionally retained behavior
* The symptoms become evident before the age of 5
* The child has reached a level of development that enables selective formation attachments with caregivers develop as normal, which usually occurs at the age of 1 or a developmental age – at least 9 months.
* Abnormal attachment behavior is not better accounted for by Autism Spectrum Disorder
* Abnormal attachment behavior is not limited to a specific dyadic relationship.

Disinhibited Social Engagement Disorder
A history of insufficient care of a child may include:
* Persistent disregard for the child's basic emotional (comfort, progress, feelings) and physical needs
* Many new caregivers (e.g. repeated changes in foster care providers)
* Upbringing in an unusual conditions (e.g. institutions) that preclude the formation of stable selective attachments
* Bullying
* Constant pattern of clearly abnormal child social behaviors – reduced or absent restraint in approaching and interacting with strangers adults, including at least one of the following:
  * Excessively familiar behavior with unknown adults, including verbal or physical
  * infringement of socially appropriate physical and verbal boundaries (seeking
  * comfort, asking age-inappropriate questions)
  * Reduced or absent contact with an adult guardian after setting off even under unknown conditions
  * A willingness to go off with an unfamiliar adult out of hand
* The symptoms are evident before the age of 5.
* The child has reached a level of development that enables selective formation attachments with caregivers develop as normal, which usually occurs at the age of 1 or a developmental age – at least 9 months.
* Abnormal attachment behavior is not better accounted for by another mental disorder (e.g. Attention Deficit Hyperactivity Disorder).

The etiological factors of attachment disorders include mental and physical neglect or abuse of a child as a result of lack of care or its inappropriate nature (a lack of response to its needs, both physical and mental, with the use of severe punishments, beatings, abuse and sometimes sexual abuse). It is worth noting that the described diagnostic criteria of attachment disorders are consistent with the description of attachment patterns in psychological theories. Both from a psychological and medical perspective, the functioning patterns based on insecure attachment styles or diagnosed attachment disorders constitute an important risk factor for mental disorders and dysfunctional interpersonal relationships in adulthood (e.g. family, peer group, work environment).

Attachment, new technologies and mental health

A literature review and experience from clinical practice of psychotherapists and psychologists emphasize the relationship between the pattern of attachment represented by a person and the pattern of pro-or anti-health behaviors related to the use of new technologies in everyday life. Media messages and new technologies are, on the one hand, a source of positive psychosocial development and pro-health behaviors, and on the other hand, social media, the Internet can be an important source of messages enhancing the development of various symptoms of mental disorders abnormal for health: anxiety, depression, addiction to psychoactive substances, personality disorders, eating disorders, etc. The influence of the media and the Internet (apart from its positive influence) on the strengthening of various mental disorders and psychoactive substance addiction syndromes, especially behavioral addictions, is becoming common. The world of the Internet and the verbal and non-verbal content of self-esteem, body image, standards determining functioning in everyday life and establishing social relations, conveyed through it, occupy a special place in the development and maintenance of mental health and its various disorders.

People with insecure attachment styles find it easier to establish relationships in the online space (Jenkins-Guarnieri and Hudibur, 2012; Trub, 2017). They can also experience a greater sense of psychological support and intimacy in this space (Nitzburg and Farber, 2013; Oldmeadow et al., 2013). These issues have already been described in more detail in Chapter 2 of this book. A review of the literature research and clinical practice of psychologists and psychotherapists often remain convergent and confirm that the pattern of attachment studied by psychological methods (Ainsworth, 1979) and subsequent attachment-related states of mind (Main et al., 1986) are important for the development of potential risk factors and protection in the context of attachment patterns (Carlson et al., 1995). However, it is very interesting, how modern technologies influence the experience of psychopoathological symptoms, as well as what their role is in shaping various types of disorders.

Contemporary mass culture and the related strong internalization of socio-cultural standards promoted by social media affect the development of self-image, self-esteem, various emotions, thoughts and human behavior: from overly submissive or perfectionist behavior (excessively subordinate to social standards) to various self-destructive behaviors: overt (suicide attempts, self-harm, anorexic behavior related to negation of one's own body) and indirect self-destructive behavior (compulsive behavior and addictions, for example, overeating, bulimic behavior, gambling, Internet addiction, for example computer games or problematic binge-watching) (Starosta et al., 2019; 2020; Izydorczyk and Sitnik-Warchulska, 2018).

New technologies and socio-cultural standards of contemporary body beauty

The ideal image of a beautiful body, promoted with the use of new technologies: the Internet and social media, has a special place in contemporary mass culture. By design, it influences the attractiveness and success in life. The self-esteem of the body is a psychological variable in a special and common way subjected to socio-cultural influence, which is reflected, for example, in the increasingly common phenomena of westernization and sexualization in the approach to the body image (Fredrickson and Roberts, 1997). As confirmed by the literature review, the mass media, social forums and the Internet often focus on communicating and promoting the universal ideal image of an attractive body figure of a woman and a man (Gültzow et al., 2020; Monks et al., 2021). The intensity and universality of the impact of new technologies and socio-cultural standards transmitted by new technologies and sociocultural standards support the pursuit of excessive body thinness and the fulfillment of socio-cultural standards of body attractiveness and promotes the development and consolidation of negative self-esteem in both men and women (Pope et al., 2000; Rollero, 2012; Zurbriggen et al., 2011).

Supported by the sociocultural standards of body beauty present in social media, the process of westernization is associated with the increasingly common phenomenon of objectification (sexualization) of the female body and, more and more, of the male body (Fredrickson and Roberts, 1997; Rollero, 2012). This phenomenon affects different cultures. As evidenced by the research conducted by the authors of this book, they take different specifics depending on the country and cultural context. For example, Asian women seem less satisfied with their appearance than European (Polish) women. However, they have a lower level of preoccupation with being overweight and fear of obesity (Izydorczyk et al., 2020; 2021).

Increasingly, it is also observed in contemporary mass culture (the Internet) standards promoting the importance of having a "sculpted", athletic body musculature, similar to that of an athlete. Internalizing the ideal of an athletic body can be as harmful as internalizing the ideal of a lean body. This, in turn, may be associated with effects such as eating disorders (Bell et al., 2016), excessive exercise (Donovan et al., 2020; Hofman, 2010), objectification (Betz and Ramsey, 2017), and self-body dissatisfaction (Donovan et al., 2020). On the one hand, the global development of new technologies is a factor contributing to the internalization of the promoted sociocultural standards of a beautiful, attractive female and male body, regardless of their nationality and place of residence. On the other hand, the widespread availability of new technologies in social life and upbringing from an early age is called a universal factor influencing the development of human mental resources (mental resilience, personality maturity, especially the attachment pattern and building emotional relationships with other people). To sum up, the socio-cultural impact of the Internet in promoting standards can be both positive and negative, supporting or limiting a person's ability to build self-esteem (including body self-esteem), consolidate safe (trustful, meeting the needs of social contact) or insecure (distrustful of people) pattern of emotional relationship.

Attachment, new technologies and addictions

The emerging scientific interest in the issue of the relationship between attachment patterns and attachment needs in adulthood draws the attention of researchers to the problems of emotional self-regulation in the group of patients addicted to various psychoactive substances (Rick and Vanheule, 2007; Schindler, 2019; Wedekind et al., 2013). The analysis of research shows that insecure attachment patterns increase the risk of developing broadly understood psychopathology during life and that it is worth taking into account the thesis that addiction to alcohol or other psychoactive substances may constitute a secondary disorder in relation to attachment disorders (Wyrzykowska et al., 2014). Many scientific studies indicate that in the group of patients addicted to alcohol and other psychoactive substances, people with insecure attachment styles dominate, including an intense pattern of attachment based on fear and avoidance (Thorberg and Lyvers, 2006; Wedekind et al., 2013) and associated with the presence of features of depression (Wedekind et al., 2013), schizoidism and alexithymia (Rick and Vanheule, 2007; Thorberg et al., 2011). People addicted to alcohol are significantly less likely to show a pattern of trusting attachment to people. They experience distrust and fear more often in interpersonal relationships, and avoid closeness and intimacy. People with disorganized attachment may abuse substances to minimize social anxiety for coping with anxiety and posttraumatic stress symptoms. People with the avoidance-type attachment pattern may abuse substances to reduce their feelings of negative emotions, attachment needs and feelings of loneliness. From an attachment theory perspective, substance abuse can be understood as "self-medication" as an attempt to compensate for the lack of effective attachment strategies (Schindler, 2019).

Reviews of contemporary research on the relationship between attachment and addiction mainly concern addiction to psychoactive substances. However, there is a lack of research analyzing the topic of the relationship between attachment and behavioral addictions. This does not mean, however, that this type of relationship is not observed in clinical practice, especially in the era of ubiquitous technology.

In the group of difficulties in which information and communication technology plays a key role as a risk factor and a trigger, disorders such as binge watching and excessive playing of computer games or dependence on operating on streaming platforms or, in fact, video games are beginning to appear. Using such forms of activity, of course, is not directly burdened with negative consequences. On the one hand, such activities can build and support the psychosocial development of modern people. On the other hand, they can also be a symptom of abnormal health behaviors that resemble behavioral addictive behaviors. The phenomenon of over-realizing emotional needs through the virtual world and using it to regulate affect is characteristic of behavioral addictions (Kim, 2019; Sprong, 2019). The specific features of behavioral addiction are often: loss of self-control, rush, regret, neglect of duties, negative social relationships and health consequences, lying, and even withdrawal symptoms such as anxiety, nervousness, rage and difficulty concentrating.

It is also worth noting that the use of binge-watching behaviors or reaching for computer games in everyday life is now common. There is therefore a clear difficulty in defining the boundary between the normal and unhealthy level of severity and frequency of this type of behavior. Another problem is to what extent reaching for this type of activity is consciously controlled. Consequently, it is difficult to precisely determine to what extent people abuse the Internet, play computer games, watch TV series, etc., and to what extent they only prefer this type of activity compared to other forms in everyday life. Perhaps it would be appropriate to consider this type of behavior as a dimension where one extreme would be the episodic use of this type of activity, and the other extreme would be to seek this type of activity in a way that is characteristic of symptoms of addiction (abuse without conscious control and using it to regulate emotional states such as such as fear, anxiety, depressed mood, feeling lonely or others). Thus, binge watching or computer games may constitute an element of the typical functioning of modern, hybrid generations. They can also, in extremes, favor and strengthen the insecure pattern of a person's emotional relationships, especially when there is a loss of control over their use.

Binge watching behaviors – between health and behavioral addiction

Binge-watching, through a system of behaviors that usually consists of watching serials, is a psychological phenomenon involving both the spectrum of positive and negative emotional reactions. At the same time, it engages a person's various cognitive processes (perception, memory, attention, thinking). Both the emotions experienced by a person during binge-watching and cognitive processes that may result in excessive loss of control over the number of watched episodes (Schweidel and Moe, 2016; Granow et al., 2018; Flayelle et al., 2019; Flayelle, 2020).

Binge-watching behaviors refer not only to watching TV series on the Internet and streaming platforms but are also related to the entire lifestyle, including establishing and shaping interpersonal relationships. They can be used not only for entertainment and health-promoting, but binge watching can also meet the criteria of behaviors and symptoms typical of behavioral addiction (Orosz et al., 2016; Trouleau, 2016; Flayelle, 2020; Starosta et al., 2020). The development of streaming platforms for watching movies and series allows a person to watch materials at a convenient time and without advertising breaks. Universal access to the use of social media, internet platforms, TV programs changes viewers' behavior while watching. The intensely growing popularity of the series and the various platforms on which they can be watched made it one of the most popular forms of spending time. In fact, we can risk a statement that following the fate of popular movie characters has become a trend in subsequent episodes and seasons. It is also a frequent element of discussions during social meetings or activities around which family life focuses. Binge-watching has thus become a way of satisfying many everyday human needs.

A research review shows that the most common motivations for binge-watching behavior are entertainment and relaxation. Panda and Pandey (2017) emphasize the presence of strong social motivation in people who reveal binge-watching behaviors too often. Many studies emphasize the use of binge-watching behaviors as a strategy of regulating one's emotions and dealing with negative affective states. Binge-watching behavior may also result from the desire to "escape" from experiencing difficult, negative emotions and from solving difficult situations. People with a strong need to use binge-watching behaviors tend to binge watching in order to escape reality, which may result in limiting the use of other, more adaptive ways of dealing with negative emotions (Panda and Pandey, 2017).

The widespread availability of online series on streaming platforms makes them easy to access. As a consequence, it can amplify the loss of control over the amount of screen time spent in front of you. As a rule, the following sections are arranged in such a way that it is easy to automatically start the next one. Their diversity, also increasing attention to quality and details, invites you to immerse yourself in the virtual world. This fosters the tendency to meet emotional needs online, which may result in the development of anti-health/pro-health behaviors (Orosz, 2016; Chambliss, 2017; Exelmans, 2017; Riddle, 2017; Flayelle, 2019).

Binge-watching behaviors may not be beneficial to health by meeting the criteria of behavioral addiction to the Internet or the criteria of addiction to video games (WHO, 2019). There are some similarities between addiction to new technologies and excessive binge-watching. A literature review and the experience from clinical practice of psychologists and psychotherapists indicate that binge-watching behaviors bearing the features of behavioral addiction (problematic binge watching) are partially justified by human personality traits, ways of regulating affect and the motivation manifested by the individual (Flayelle, 2019; Flayelle, 2020; Starosta and Izydorczyk, 2020). Many studies on the issue of behavioral addictions indicate a relationship between problematic use and anxiety and depression (Mehroof, 2010; Van Rooij et al., 2014; Liu et al., 2018). The problematic use of social media or video games, as well as psychoactive substances, can be used to regulate affect by anxious and depressive persons in order to obtain positive gratification and protect themselves from negative feelings (Cheetham, 2010; Nikmanesh et al., 2014). A review of many studies shows the relationship between the frequency of binge-watching behaviors and depression, a sense of alienation and loneliness (Ahmed, 2017; Flayelle, 2019; Sun and Chang, 2021; Steins-Loeber et al. 2020; Wheeler, 2015). These symptoms are undoubtedly associated with disturbances in emotional regulation, binge watching may be a means to regulate them, at least temporarily, thus favoring the development of a tendency to become addicted to watching serials.

Other research shows that binge watching, moving towards instant gratification and emotional regulation, is a maladaptive coping strategy, as is problematic internet/computer use, gambling and social media addiction. Thus, the motivation for binge-watching behaviors can be varied: from regulating emotions to satisfying many other needs and goals, such as positive affect, entertainment, relaxation and social relations (Panda and Pandey 2017; Rubenking and Bracken, 2018). Other factors motivating binge watching are cognitive motivation – seeking information (Starosta et al., 2019; Shimand Kim, 2018), the need to deal with loneliness, the need to avoid duties and difficulties in carrying out tasks (Tóth-Király et al., 2017). We can also talk about the "escape" motivation in the development of binge watching behaviors, which allows an individual to escape from problems and regulate negative (also impulsive) emotions (Panda and Pandey, 2017; Rubenking and Bracken, 2018; Flayelle, 2019; Starosta et al., 2019). We can therefore wonder to what extent highly impulsive people will more often than others represent an insecure pattern of attachment, which may help to relieve emotional tensions and regulate experienced emotions through the use of binge watching behaviors. These behaviors, as socially acceptable and difficult to define, may in some way help protect the ego, or at least not violate it too much.

The virtual world of computer games and mental health

Among the new technologies present in the everyday life of a human being, attention is drawn to the widespread use of computer games by people who also present various patterns of attachment and building interpersonal relationships. It can be assumed that some people, probably with a secure attachment style, will use the virtual world in a way that we would call health-promoting. People with insecure attachment style will probably present anti-health behaviors (Internet addiction, abuse of computer games) in the use of modern information and communication technologies.

When analyzing the impact of computer games on mental health and the emerging emotional and social disorders, both positive and negative effects should be taken into account. A research review and clinical practice confirm that the excessive use of computer games is often associated with a decrease in psychophysical well-being (Hagström and Kaldo, 2014), with an increase in emotional disorders: anxiety, social phobia, aggression, depression, social alienation and symptoms of behavioral addiction among children and adults (Colder- Carras et al., 2018; Mentozoni et al., 2011; Mérelle et al., 2017, Gonzáles-Bueso et al., 2018) or an increase in excessive fatigue, attention and sleep disorders and social functioning disorders (Mandryk and Birk, 2017; Saquib et al., 2017, Wartberg et al., 2019). Some studies indicate that people addicted to social media are more likely to abuse alcohol (Rikkers et al., 2016), present suicide attempts (Lee et al., 2017), exhibit depressive symptoms and obsessive-compulsive disorders (Stockdale and Coyne, 2018). Some studies have indicated that depression and loneliness are associated with pathological playing of computer games (Krossbakken et al., 2018). Computer games can also be a kind of "escape from problems" mechanism (Hrafnkelsdottir et al., 2018; Taheri et al., 2018). They can also be associated with depression and anxiety. On the one hand, depression and anxiety may be the cause of excessive use of computer games and, on the other hand, depression and anxiety can result from gaming addiction.

However, in the everyday life of modern people, the use of computer games is not always anti-health. In many situations, the virtual world of computer games is a factor influencing health-promoting behaviors, serving the development and maintenance of mental well-being. Playing computer games or video games can be a source of strengthening mental well-being, correcting the mood and reducing the level of perceived distress, enhancing the sense of relaxation and positive ways of coping with stress. It can also promote proper emotional regulation (Villani et al., 2018), have a positive effect on mental health (Fleming et al., 2017) and on the functioning of cognitive processes, such as concentration and creativity. It can also motivate to act and make social contacts, especially among adolescents (Ferguson and Olson, 2013). After all, the virtual world in computer games can be used in the process of psychological therapy (most often in the behavioral-cognitive paradigm) in many people suffering from phobia, anxiety and depression (Colder Carras et al., 2018; Fish et al., 2018), PTSD (Botella, et al., 2015), in psychological treatment of children with attention deficit hyperactivity disorder (Bul et al., 2016), or in the treatment of children and adolescents with anxiety symptoms (Scholten, 2016; Wols et al., 2018).

Summarizing the content in this chapter, it is worth emphasizing that the patterns of early childhood bonds along with safe or insecure patterns of establishing emotional relationships in adulthood, shaped by many psychosocial factors (including new technologies), constitute an important risk factor for the

Table 4.2 The pattern of bonding a person and the basic psychological reactions related to the use of new technologies in everyday life

Pattern of attachment	Characteristics of psychological indicators in the context of using modern technologies in everyday life
Safe attachment	A pattern of emotional and interpersonal relationships based on empathy and the ability to understand the internal experiences of other people; the preserved ability to establish and maintain an emotional bond with other people; the ability to self-reflection provide the basis for a correct (healthy) response to new technologies and their application in a person's life. No increased tendencies towards behavioral addictions. Positive influence of games and the Internet on mental development
Anxiety-avoiding attachment	A pattern of emotional and interpersonal relationships based on the maintained distrust, limitations and lack of flexibility in establishing emotional and social relationships, strong anxiety motivation to act, which gives grounds for using new technologies as a way of anxious and depressive solutions to difficult situations and emotional tensions
Ambivalent attachment	A pattern of emotional and interpersonal relationships based on distrust, limitations in the ability to understand other people's internal experiences and the ability to maintain emotional ties, and limited ability to self-reflect and understand other people's internal experiences. New technologies (the Internet, computer games) can be a source of behaviors aimed at discharging, reducing emotional tensions, aggression, the tendency to reveal personality disorders and behavioral and other addictions
Disorganized attachment	Pattern of emotional and interpersonal relationship based on strong distrust, limitations and lack of flexibility in establishing emotional and social relationships, emotional lability, self-destructive behavior. Occurrence of mental disorders based on the disintegration of the personality structure at the borderline and psychotic level. New technologies (the Internet, computer games, binge watching) are a source of self-destructive, impulsive behaviors related mainly to personality disorders, tendency to behavioral and other addictions

development of pro-health or unhealthy behaviors and mental disorders. The potential relationship between individual attachment patterns and the propensity to use technology in a risky, anti-health and disease context is presented in Table 4.2.

References

Ahmed, A.A.M. (2017). New Era of TV-Watching Behavior: Binge Watching and its Psychological Effect. *Media Watch*, 8(2), 192–207. DOI: 10.15655/mw/2017/v8i2/49006

Ainsworth, M.S. (1979). Infant–mother attachment. *American Psychologist*, 34(10), 932–937. DOI: 10.1037/0003-066X.34.10.932

Bamford, B., Halliwell, E. (2009). Investigating the role of attachment in social comparison theories of eating disorders within a non-clinical female population. *European Eating Disorders Review*, 17(5), 371–379. DOI: 10.1002/erv.951, indexed in Pubmed: 19593745.

Beeney, J.E., Stepp, S.D., Hallquist, M.N., (2015). Attachment and social cognition in borderline personality disorder: Specificity in relation to antisocial and avoidant personality disorders. *Personal Disorders*, 6(3), 207–215. DOI: 10.1037/per0000110, indexed in Pubmed: 25705979.

Bell, H.S., Donovan, C.L., Ramme, R. (2016). Is athletic really ideal? An examination of the mediating role of body dissatisfaction in predicting disordered eating and compulsive exercise. *Eating Behaviors*, 21, 24–26. DOI: 10.1016/j.eatbeh.2015.12.012

Betz, D.E., Ramsey, L.R. (2017). Should women be "All About That Bass?": Diverse body-ideal messages and women's body image. *Body Image*, 22, 18–31. DOI: 10.1016/j.bodyim.2017.04.004

Bifulco, A., Kwon, J., Jacobs, C., Moran, P.M., Bunn, A., Beer, N. (2006). Styl przywiązania dorosłych jako mediator między zaniedbaniem/nadużyciem w dzieciństwie a depresją i lękiem u dorosłych. *Social Psychiatry and Psychiatric Epidemiology*, 41, 796–805. pmid:16871369

Boldrini, T., Pontillo, M., Tanzilli, A., Giovanardi, G., Di Cicilia, G., Salcuni, S., Vicari, S., Lingiardi, V. (2020a). An attachment perspective on the risk for psychosis: Clinical correlates and the predictive value of attachment patterns and mentalization. *Schizofrenia Research*, DOI: 10.1016/j.schres.2020.05.052

Boldrini, T., Tanzilli, A., Di Gualco, C.I., Lingiardi, V., Salcuni, S., Tata, M.K., Vicari, S., Pontillo, M. (2020b). Personality Traits and Disorders in Adolescents at Clinical High Risk for Psychosis: Toward a Clinically Meaningful Diagnosis. *Frontiers in Psychiatry*, 11(8). DOI: 10.3389/fpsyt.2020.562835

Botella, C., Serrano, B., Baños, R.M., Garcia-Palacios, A. (2015). Virtual reality exposure-based therapy for the treatment of post-traumatic stress disorder: a review of its efficacy, the adequacy of the treatment protocol, and its acceptability. *Neuropsychiatric Disease and Treatment*, 11, 2533–2545. DOI: 10.2147/NDT.S89542

Bul, K.C.M., Kato, P.M., Van der Oord, S., Danckaerts, M., Vreeke, L.J., Willems, A., Van Oers, H.J.J., Van Den Heuvel, R., Birnie, D., Van Amelsvoort, T.A.M.J., Franken, I. H. A., Maras, A. (2016). Behavioral Outcome Effects of Serious Gaming as an Adjunct to Treatment for Children With Attention-Deficit. Hyperactivity Disorder: A Randomized Controlled Trial. *Journal of Medical Internet Research*, 18(2), 26. DOI: 10.2196/jmir5173

Carlson, E., Sroufe, L.A. (1995). Contributions of attachment theory to developmental psychopathology. In: D. Cicchetti, D. J. Cohen (Eds.). *Developmental Psychopathology*, (pp. 581–617) New York, Wiley.

Carr, S.C.H., Hardy, A., Fornells-Ambrojo, M. (2018). Relationship between attachment style and symptom severity across the psychosis spectrum: A meta-analysis. *Clinical Psychology Review*, 59, 145–158. DOI: 10.1016/j.cpr.2017.12.001

Chambliss, C., Gartenberg, C., Honrychs, D., Elko, M., Match, R., McGill, S., Watters, M., Bayer, K., Boylan, C., Hanson, A. (2017). Distracted by Binge-watching: Sources of

Academic and Social Disruption in Students. *ARC Journal of Pediatrics*, 3, 14–17. DOI: 10.20431/2455-5711.0301004

Chatziioannidis, S., Andreou, Ch., Agorastos, A., Kaprinis, S., Malliaris, Y., Garyfallos, G., Bozikas, V. (2019). The role of attachment anxiety in the relationship between childhood trauma and schizophrenia-spectrum psychosis. *Psychiatry Research*, 276, 223–231. DOI: 10.1016/j.psychres.2019.05.021

Cheetham, A., Allen, N.B., Yücel, M., Lubman, D.I. (2010). The role of affective dysregulation in drug addiction. *Clinical Psychology Review*, 30, 621–634. DOI: 10.1016/j.cpr.2010.04.005

Clarkin, J.F., Fonagy, P., Gabbard, G.O. (2013). *Psychoterapia psychodynamiczna zaburzeń osobowości*, Wydawnictwo Uniwersytetu Jagiellońskiego.

Colder Carras, M., Van Rooij, A.J., Spruijt-Metz, D., Kvedar, J., Griffiths, M., Carabas, Y., Labrique, A. (2018). Commercial Video Games As Therapy: A New Research Agenda to Unlock the Potential of a Global Pastime. *Frontiers in Psychiatry*, 8, 300. DOI: 10.3389/fpsyt.2017.00300

Debbané, M., Salaminios G, Luyten P., Badoud, D., Armando, M., Tozzi, S.A., Fonagy, P., Brent, K.B. (2016). Attachment, neurobiology, and mentalizing along the psychosis continuum. *Frontiers in Human Neuroscience*, 10, 406. DOI: 10.3389/fnhum.2016.00406

Donovan, C.L., Uhlmann, L.R., Loxton, N.J. (2020). Strong is the New Skinny, but is it Ideal?: A Test of the Tripartite Influence Model using a new Measure of Fit-Ideal Internalisation. *Body Image*, 35, 171–180. DOI: 10.1016/j.bodyim.2020.09.002

Eggert, J., Levendosky, A., Klump, K. (2007). Relationships among attachment styles, personality characteristics, and disordered eating. *International Journal of Eating Disorders*, 40(2), 149–155. DOI: 10.1002/eat.20351, indexed in Pubmed: 17089415.

Exelmans, L., Van den Bulck, J. (2017). Binge-Viewing, Sleep, and the Role of Pre-Sleep Arousal. *Journal of Clinical Sleep Medicine*, 13, 1001–1008. DOI: 10.5664/jcsm.6704

Ferguson, Ch.J., Olson, Ch.K. (2013). Friends, fun, frustration and fantasy: Child motivations for video game play. *Motivation and Emotion*, 37(1), 154–164.

Fish, M., Russoniello, C., O'Brien, K. (2018). Zombies vs. Anxiety: An Augmentation Study of Prescribed Video Game Play Compared to Medication in Reducing Anxiety Symptoms. *Simulation & Gaming*, 49(5), 553–566. DOI: 10.1177/1046878118773126

Flayelle, M., Maurage, P., Di Lorenzo, R.K., Vögele G.S.M., Billieux, J. (2020). Binge-watching: What do we know so far? A first systematic review of the evidence. *Current Addiction Reports*, 7, 44–60. DOI: 10.1007/s40429-020-00299-8

Flayelle, M., Maurage, P., Karila, L., Claus, V., Billieux, J. (2019). Overcoming the unitary exploration of binge-watching: A cluster analytical approach. *Journal of Behavioral Addictions*, 8, 586–602. DOI: 10.1556/2006.8.2019.53

Fleming, T.M., Bavin, L., Stasiak, K., Hermansson-Webb, E., Merry S.N., Cheek, C.M., Ho M.L., Pollmuller, B., Hetrick, S. (2017). Serious Games and Gamification for Mental Health: Current Status and Promising Directions. *Frontiers in Psychiatry*. DOI: 10.3389/fpsyt.2016.00215

Fredrickson, B.L., Roberts, T.A. (1997). Objectification theory. Toward understanding women's lived experiences and mental health risks. *Psychology of Women Quarterly*, 21, 173–206. DOI: 10.1111/j.1471-6402.1997.tb00108.x

Gabbard, G. (2013). *Psychoterapia psychodynamiczna zaburzeń osobowości. Podręcznik kliniczny*, Kraków: Wydawnictwo Uniwersytetu Jagiellońskiego, ISBN 978-83-233-3448-4

Gabbard, G. (2015). *Psychiatra psychodynamiczna w praktyce klinicznej*. Kraków: Wydawnictwo Uniwersytetu Jagiellońskiego, ISBN 978-83-233-3917-5

Gonzáles-Bueso, V., Santamaria, J.J., Fernandéz, D., Merino, L., Montero, E., Ribas, J. (2018). International Journal of Environmental Research and Public Health, 15(6), 668. DOI: 10.3390/ijerph15040668

Granow, V., Reinecke, L., Ziegele, M. (2018). Binge-watching & psychological wellbeing: Media use between lack of control and perceived autonomy. *Communication Research Reports*, 35(5), 392–401. DOI: 10.1080/08824096.2018.1525347

Green, J.G, McLaughlin, K.A., Berglund, P.A. (2010). Childhood adversities and adult psychiatric disorders in the national comorbidity survey replication I: associations with first onset of DSM-IV disorders. *Archives of General Psychiatry*, 67(2), 113–123, DOI: 10.1001/archgenpsy-chiatry.2009.186, indexed in Pubmed: 20124111.

Gültzow, T., Guidry, J.P.D., Schneider, F., Hoving, C. (2020). Male body image portrayals on Instagram. *Cyberpsychology, Behavior and Social Networking*, 23, 281–289. DOI: 10.1089/cyber.2019.0368

Hagström, D., Kaldo, Viktor (2014). Escapism Among Players of MMORPGs—Conceptual Clarification, Its Relation to Mental Health Factors, and Development of a New Measure. *Cyberpsychology, Behavior, and Social Networking*, 17, 19–25. DOI: 10.1089/cyber.2012.0222

Hofman, K. (2010). Athletic-ideal and thin-ideal internalization as prospective predictors of body dissatisfaction, dieting, and compulsive exercise. *Body Image*, 7(3), 240–245. DOI: 10.1016/j.bodyim.2010.02.004

Hrafnkelsdottir, S.M., Brychta, R.J., Rognvaldsdottir, V., Gestsdottir, S., Chen, K.Y., Johannsson, E., Guðmundsdottir, S.L., Arngrimsson, S.A. (2018). Less screen time and more frequent vigorous physical activity is associated with lower risk of reporting negative mental health symptoms among Icelandic adolescents. *PLoS One*, 13(4). DOI: 10.1371/journal.pone.0196286

Izydorczyk, B., Sitnik-Warchulska, K. (2018). Sociocultural Appearance Standards and Risk Factors for Eating Disorders in Adolescents and Women of Various Ages. *Frontiers in Psychology*, 29(9), 429. DOI: 10.3389/fpsyg.2018.00429

Izydorczyk, B., Truong, T.K.H., Lipowska, M., Sitnik-Warchulska, K., Lizińczyk, S. (2021). Psychological Risk Factors for the Development of Restrictive and Bulimic Eating Behaviors: A Polish and Vietnamese Comparison. *Nutrients*, 13(3), 910. DOI: 10.3390/nu13030910

Izydorczyk, B., Truong, T.K.H., Lizińczyk, S., Sitnik-Warchulska, K., Lipowska, M., Gulbicka, A. (2020). Body Dissatisfaction, Restrictive, and Bulimic Behaviours Among Young Women: A Polish-Japanese Comparison. *Nutrients*, 12(3), 666. DOI: 10.3390/nu12030666

Jenkins-Guarnieri, M.A., Wright, S.L., Hudiburgh, L.M. (2012). The relationships among attachment style, personality traits, interpersonal competency, and Facebook use. *Journal of Applied Developmental Psychology*, 33(6), 294–301. DOI: 10.1016/j.appdev.2012.08.001

Kim, S. (2019). Workaholism, Motivation, and Addiction in the Workplace: A Critical Review and Implications for HRD. *Human Resource Development Review*, 18(3), 325–348. DOI: 10.1177/1534484319845164

Kochanska, G., Kim, S. (2012). Toward a new understanding of legacy of early attachments for future antisocial trajectories: evidence from two longitudinal studies. *Development and Psychopathology*, 24(3), 783–806. DOI: 10.1017/S0954579412000375

Korver-Nieberg, N., Berry, K., Meijer, C.J., de Haan, L. (2014). Adult attachment and psychotic phenomenology in clinical and non-clinical samples: a systematic review. *Psychology and Psychotherapy*, 87(2), 127–154. DOI: 10.1111/papt.12010

Krawczyk, P., Święcicki, Ł. (2020). ICD-11 vs. ICD-10 – przegląd aktualizacji i nowości wprowadzonych w najnowszej wersji Międzynarodowej Klasyfikacji Chorób WHO ICD-11 vs. ICD-10 – [a review of updates and novelties introduced in the latest version of the WHO International Classification of Diseases], *Psychiatria Polska*, 54(1), 7–20. www.psychiatriapolska.pl. DOI: 10.12740/PP/103876

Krossbakken, E., Pallessen, S., Mentzoni, R.A., King, D.L., Molde, H.M., Finserås, T.R., Toshemi, T. (2018). A Cross-Lagged Study of Developmental Trajectories of Video Game Engagement, Addiction, and Mental Health. *Frontiers in Psychology*, 9, 2239. DOI: 10.3389/fpsyg.2018.02239

Lavin, R., Bucci, S., Varese, F., Berry, K. (2020). The relationship between insecure attachment and paranoia in psychosis: A systematic literature review. *British Journal of Clinical Psychology*, 59(1), 39–65. DOI: 10.1111/bjc.12231

Lee, H. H., Sung, J. H., Lee, J. Y., Lee, J. E. (2017). Differences by Sex in Association of Mental Health with Video Gaming or Other Nonacademic Computer Use Among US Adolescents. *Preventing Chronic Disease*, 14, 117. DOI: 10.5888/pcd14.170151

Liu, L., Yao, Y.W., Li, C.R., Zhang, J.T., Xia, C.C., Lan, J.T. (2018). The comorbidity between internet gaming disorder and depression: interrelationship and neural mechanisms. *Frontiers in Psychiatry*, 9, 154. DOI: 10.3389/fpsyt.2018.00154

Llewellyn-Jones, S., Perez, J., Cano-Domínguez, P., de-Luis-Matilla, A., Espina-Eizaguirre, A., Reneses, B., Ochoa, S.C. (2019). Clinical personality traits and parental bonding in patients with recent onset of psychosis. *Schizophrenia Research*, 212, 237–238. DOI: 10.1016/j.schres.2019.07.052

Main, M., Solomon, J. (1986). Discovery of an insecure-disorganized/disoriented attachment pattern. W: T. B. Brazelton, M. W. Yogman, (Eds.) *Affective Development in Infancy*. (pp. 95–124), Westport, CT, US: Ablex Publishing.

Mandryk, R.L., Birk, M.V. (2017). Toward Game-Based Digital Mental Health Interventions: Player Habits and Preferences. *Journal of Medical Internet Research*, 19(4), 128. DOI: 10.2196/jmir/6906

Mehroof, M., Griffiths, M.D. (2010). Online gaming addiction: The role of sensation seeking, self-control, neuroticism, aggression, state anxiety, and trait anxiety. *Cyberpsychology & Behavior*, 13, 313–316.

Mentozoni R.A., Brunborg, G. S., Molde, H., Myrseth, H., Skouverøe, Hetland, J, & Pallesen, S. (2011). Problematic vide game use: estimated prevelance and associations with mental and physical health. *Cyberpsychology, Behavior and Social Networking*. 14(10), 591–596. DOI: 10.1089/cyber.2010.0260

Mérelle, S.Y.M., Kleiboer, A.M., Schotanus, M., Cluitmans, T.L.M., Waardenburg, C.M., Kramer, D., Can de Mheen, D., Van Rooij, A.J. (2017). Which health-related problems areassociated with problematic video-gaming or social media use in adolescents? A large scale cross-sectional study. *Clinical Neuropsychiatry*, 14(1), 11–19.

Mikulincer, M., Florian, V. (1998). The relationship between adult attachment styles and emotional and cognitive reactions to stressful events. In: J. A. Simpson, W. S. Rholes, (Eds.) *Attachment Theory and Close Relationships*. (pp. 143–165), New York: Guilford Press.

Mikulincer, M. (1998b). Adult attachment style and individual differences in functional versus dysfunctional experiences of anger. *Journal of Personality and Social Psychology*, 74(2), 513–524.

Mikulincer, M., Shaver, P.R. (2010). Attachment bases of psychopathology. In: M. Mikulincer, P. R. Shaver, (Eds.). *Attachment in Adulthood. Structure, Dynamics, Change*. (pp. 369–404), New York/London: The Guilford Press.

Monks, H., Costello, L., Dare, J., Boyd, E.R. (2021). We're continually comparing ourselves to something: Navigating body image, media, and social media ideals at the nexus of appearance, health, and wellness. *Sex Roles*, 84, 221–237. DOI: 10.1007/s11199-020-01162

Murphy, R., Goodall, K., Woodrow, A. (2020). The relationship between attachment insecurity and experiences on the paranoia continuum: A meta-analysis. *British Journal of Clinical Psychology*, 59(3), 290–318. DOI: 10.1111/bjc.12247

Myers, S.G., Wells, A. (2015). Early trauma, negative affect, and anxious attachment: the role of metacognition. *Anxiety Stress Coping*, 28(6), 634–649. DOI: 10.1080/10615806.2 015.1009832

Nitzburg, G.C., Farber, B.A. (2013). Putting up emotional (Facebook) walls? Attachment status and emerging adults' experiences of social networking sites. *Journal of Clinical Psychology*, 69(11), 1183–1190. DOI: 10.1002/jclp.22045

Nikmanesh, Z., Kazemi, Y., Khosravy, M. (2014). Study role of different dimensions of emotional self-regulation on addiction potential. *Journal of Family & Reproductive Health*, 8(2), 69–72.

Oldmeadow, J.A., Quinn, S., Kowert, R. (2013). Attachment style, social skills, and Facebook use amongst adults. *Computers in Human Behavior*, 29(3), 1142–1149. DOI: 10.1016/j.chb.2012.10.006

Orosz, G., Bőthe, B., Tóth-Király, I. (2016). The development of the Problematic Series WatchingScale (PSWS). *Journal of Behavioral Addictions*, 5(1), 144–150. DOI: 10.1556/2 006.5.2016.011

Panda, S., Pandey, S. (2017). Binge-watching and collage students: Motivations and outcomes. *Young Consumers*, 18, 425–438. DOI: 10.1108/YC-07-2017-00707

Pope, H., Gruber, A., Mangweth, B., Bureau, B., deCol, C., Jouvent, R., Hudson, J. (2000). Body image perception among men in three countries. *American Journal of Psychiatry*, 157(8), 1297–1301. DOI: 10.1176/appi.ajp.157.8.1297

Ramos, V., Canta, G., de Castro, F. (2016). The relation between attachment, personality, internalizing, and externalizing dimensions in adolescents with borderline personality disorder. *Bulletin of the Menninger Clinic*, 80(3), 213–233, DOI: 10.1521/bumc.2016.80.3.213

Rick, A., Vanheule, S. (2007). Attachment styles in alcoholic inpatients. *European Addiction Research*, 13(2), 101–108. DOI: 10.1159/000097940

Riem, M.M., Bakermans-Kranenburg, M.J., van IJzendoorn, M.H., Out, D., Rombouts, S.A. (2012). Attachment in the brain: adult attachment representations predict amygdala and behavioral responses to infant crying. *Attachment & Human Development*, 14(6), 533–551. DOI: 10.1080/14616734.2012.727252. PMID: 23106177

Riddle, K., Peebles, A., Davis, C., Xu, F., Schroeder, E. (2017). The Addictive Potential of Television Binge Watching: Comparing Intentional and Unintentional Binges. *Psychology of Popular Media Culture*, 7. DOI: 10.1037/ppm0000167

Rikkers, W., Lawrence, D., Hafekost, J., Zubrick, S.R. (2016). Internet use and electronic gaming by children and adolescents with emotional and behavioural problem in Australia –

result from the second Child and Adolescent Survey of Mental Health and Wellbeing. *BMC Public Health*, 16, 399. DOI: 10.1186/s12889-016-3058-1

Rokita, K.I., Dauvermann, M., Donohoe, G. (2018). Early life experiences and social cognition in major psychiatric disorders: A systematic review. *European Psychiatry*, 53. DOI: 10.1016/j.eurpsy.2018.06.006

Rollero, Ch. (2012). Men and women facing objectification: The effects of media models on well-being, self-esteem and ambivalent sexism. *International Journal of Social Psychology*, 28(3), 373-382. DOI: 10.1174/021347413807719166

Rubenking, B., Bracken, C.C. (2018). Binge-watching: A suspenseful, emotional habit. *Communication Research Reports*, 35, 1–11. DOI: 10.1080/08824096.2018.1525346

Saquib, N., Saquib, J., Wahid, A., Ahmed, A.A., Dhuhayr, H.E., Zaghloul, M.S., Ewid, M., Al-Mazrou, A. (2017). Video game addiction and psychological distress among expatriate adolescents in Saudi Arabia. *Addictive Behaviors Report*, 6, 12–127. DOI: 10.1016/j.abrep.2017.09.003

Schindler, A. (2019). Attachment and Substance Use Disorders—Theoretical Models, Empirical Evidence, and Implications for Treatment. *Frontiers in Psychiatry*. DOI: 10.3389/fpsyt.2019.00727

Scholten, H., Malmberg, M., Lobel, A., Engels, R.C.M.E., Granic, I. (2016). A Randomized Controlled Trial to Test the Effectiveness of an Immersive 3D Video Game for Anxiety Prevention among Adolescents. *PLoS ONE*, 11(1). DOI: 10.1371/journal.pone.0147763

Schweidel, D.A., Moe, W.W. (2016). Binge-watching and Advertising. *Journal of Marketing*, 80, 1–19. DOI: 10.1509/jm.15.0258

Sheinbaum, T., Kwapil, T.R., Barrantes-Vidal, N. (2014). Fearful attachment mediates the association of childhood trauma with schizotype and psychotic-like experiences. *Psychiatry Research*, 220(1-2), 691–693. DOI: 10.1016/j.psychres.2014.07.030

Sheinbaum, T., Bifulco, A., Ballespí, S., Mitjavila, M., Kwapil, T.E., Barrantes-Vidal, N. (2015). Interview Investigation of Insecure Attachment Styles as Mediators between Poor Childhood Care and Schizophrenia Spectrum Phenomenology. *Plos One*. DOI: 10.1371/journal.pone.0135150

Sheinbaum, T., Racioppi, A., Kwapil, T.R., Barrantes-Vidal, N. (2020). Attachment as a mechanism between childhood maltreatment and subclinical psychotic phenomena: Results from an eight-year follow-up study. *Schizophrenia Research*, 220, 261–264. DOI: 10.1016/j.schres.2020.03.023

Shim, H., Kim, K.J. (2018). An exploration of the motivations for binge-watching and the role of individual differences. *Computers in Human Behavior*, 82, 94–100. DOI: 10.1016/j.chb.2017.12.032

Sprong, M.E., Griffiths, M.D., Lloyd, D.P., Paul, E., Buono, F.D. (2019). Comparison of the Video Game Functional Assessment-Revised (VGFA-R) and Internet Gaming Disorder Test (IGD-20). *Frontiers in Psychology*, 10, 310. DOI: 10.3389/fpsyg.2019.00310

Starosta, J., Izydorczyk, B. (2020). Understanding the Phenomenon of Binge-Watching—A Systematic *Review. International Journal of Environmental Research and Public Health*, 17(4469). DOI: 10.3390/ijerph17124469

Starosta, J., Izydorczyk, B., Lizińczyk, S. (2019). Characteristics of people's binge-watching behavior in the "entering into early adulthood" period of life. *Health Psychology Report*, 7(2), 149–164. DOI: 10.5114/hpr.2019.83025

Steins-Loeber, S., Reiter, T., Averbeck, H., Harbarth, L., Brand, M. (2020). Binge-Watching Behaviour: The Role of Impulsivity and Depressive Symptoms. *European Addiction Research*, 26(3), 141-150. DOI: 10.1159/000506307

Stockdale, L., Coyne, S.M. (2018). Video game addiction in emerging adulthood: Cross-sectional evidence of pathology in video game addicts as compared to matched healthy controls. *Journal of Affective Disorders*, 225, 265–272. DOI: 10.1016/j.jad.2017.08.045

Sun, J.J., Chang, Y.J. (2021). Associations of Problematic Binge-Watching with Depression, Social Interaction Anxiety, and Loneliness. *International Journal of Environmental Researchand Public Health*, 18, 1168. DOI: 10.3390/ijerph18031168

Taheri, E., Heshmat, R., Esmaeil Motlagh, M., Adrelan, G., Asayesh, H.M., Qorbani, M., Kelishadi, R. (2018). Association of Physical Activity and Screen Time with Psychiatric Distress in Children and Adolescents: CASPIAN-IV Study. *Journal of Tropical Pediatrics*. DOI: 10.1093/tropej/fmy063

Taylor, R.E., Mann, A.H., White, N.J., Goldberg, D.P. (2000). Attachment style in patients with unexplained physical complaints. *Psychological Medicine*, 30(4), 931–941, DOI: 10.1017/s0033291799002317

Thorberg, F.A., Lyvers, M. (2006). Attachment, fear of intimacy and differentiation of self among clients in substance disorder treatment facilities. *Addictive Behaviors*, 31(4),732–773.

Thorberg, F.A., Young, E., Sullivan, K., Lyvers, M., Connor, J., Feeney, G. (2011). Alexithymia, craving and attachment in a heavy drinking population. *Addictive Behaviors*, 36(4), 427–430.DOI: 10.1016/j.addbeh.2010.12.016

Tóth-Király, I., Bőthe, B., Tóth-Fáber, E., Hága, G., Gábor, O. (2017). Connected to TV Series: Quantifying Series Watching Engagement. *Journal of Behavioral Addictions*, 6(4), 472–489.

Trouleau, W., Ashkan, A., Ding, W., Eriksson, B. (2016) Just one more: Modeling Binge Watching Behaviour. KDD '16 Proceeding of the 22nd ACM SIGKDD International Conference on Knowledge Discovery and Data Mining, Association for Computing Machinery, New York, USA, 1215–1224. DOI: 10.1145/2939672.2939792

Trub, L. (2017). A portrait of the self in the digital age: Attachment, splitting, and self-concealment in online and offline self-presentation. *Psychoanalytic Psychology*, 34(1), 78–86. DOI: 10.1037/pap0000123

Verheul, R., Andrea, H., Berghout, C.C., Dolan, C., Busschbach, J.V., van der Kroft, P.A. (2008). Severity Indices of Personality Problems (SIPP-118): development, factor structure, reliability, and validity. *Psychological Assessment*, 20, 23–34. DOI: 10.1037/1040-3590.20.1.23

Waldinger, R.J., Schulz, M.S., Barsky, A.J., Ahern, D.K. (2006). Mapping the road from childhood trauma to adult somatization: the role of attachment. *Psychosomatic Medicine*, 68(1), 129–135. DOI: 10.1097/01.psy.0000195834.37094.a4

Wartberg, L., Kriston, L., Zieglemeier, M., Lincoln, T., Kammerl, R. (2019). A longitudinal study on psychosocial causes and consequences of Internet gaming disorder in adolescence. *Psychological Medicine*, 49(20), 287–294. DOI: 10.1017/S003329171800082X

Wedekind, D., Bandelow, B., Heitmann, S., Havemann-Reinecke, U., Engel, K.R., Huether, G. (2013). Attachment style, anxiety coping, and personality-styles in withdrawn alcohol addicted inpatients.*Substance Abuse Treatment, Prevention, and Policy*, 8(1). DOI: 10.1186/1747-597X-8-1

Wheeler, K.S. (2015). *The Relationships between Television Viewing Behaviours, Attachment, Loneliness, Depression and Psychological Well-Being.* (Master Dissertation). Georgia Southern University. Available online: https://digitalcommons.georgiasouthern.edu/cgi/viewcontent.cgi?article=1142&context=honors-theses

Wols, A., Lichtwarck-Aschoff, A., Schoneveld, E. A., Granic, I. (2018). In-game Play Behaviours during an Applied Video Game for Anxiety Prevention Predict Successful Intervention Outcomes. *Journal of Psychopathology and Behavioral Assessment*, 40(4), 655–668. DOI: 10.1007/s10862-018-9684-4

World Health Organization. (2019). *Promoting Mental Health: Concepts, Emerging Evidence, Practice (Summary Report).* Geneva: World Health Organization.

World Health Organization. (2019). *ICD-11: International Classification of Diseases* (11th revision). Retrieved from https://icd.who.int/

Wyrzykowska, E., Głogowska, K., Mickiewicz, K. (2014). Relacje przywiązania u osób uzależnionych od alkoholu. *Alcoholism and Drug Addiction*, 27(2), 127–143. DOI: 10.1016/S0867-4361(14)70009-4

Van Rooij, A.J., Kuss, D.J., Griffiths, M.D., Shorter, G.W., Schoenmakers, T.M., Van De Mheen, D. (2014). The (co-) occurrence of problematic video gaming, substance use, and psychosocial problems in adolescents. *Journal of Behavioral Addiction*, 3, 157–165. DOI: 10.1556/JBA.3.2014.013

Villani, D., Carissoli, C., Triberti, S., Marchetti, A., Gilli, G., Riva, G. (2018). Videogames for Emotion Regulation: A Systematic Review. *Games for Health Journal*, 7(2), 85–99. DOI: 10.1089/g4h.2017.0108

Zachrisson, H.D., Skårderud, F. (2010). Feelings of insecurity: review of attachment and eating disorders. *European Eating Disorders Review*, 18(2), 97–106. DOI: 10.1002/erv.999.

Zurbriggen, E.L., Ramsey, L.R., Jaworski, B.K. (2011). Self- and partner-objectification in romantic relationships: associations with media consumption and relationship satisfaction. *Sex Roles*, 64, 449–462. DOI: 10.1007/s11199-011-9933-4

Żechowski, C., Cichocka, A., Rowiński, T., Mrozik, K., Kowalska-Dąbrowska, M., Czuma, I. (2018). Attachment styles and mental health of adults in generalpopulation: pilot study. *Psychiatria*, 15(4), 193–198.

Chapter 5

Contemporary trends in psychological diagnosis and assessment (online psychological diagnosis and therapy)

Attachment as an essential element of psychological diagnosis and therapy

One of the most important factors in the process of diagnosis and psychological support is the specialist's relationship with the examined person and the patient. Such a relationship in the therapeutic process is called the therapeutic relationship and is considered one of the common therapeutic factors, and according to research, this factor explains about 15% of the variance in the efficacy of psychotherapy(Norcross and Lambert, 2018). The therapeutic relationship, like many constructs in psychology and psychotherapy, is difficult to define, complex and ambiguous. One of the most popular definitions is that a therapeutic relationship is about mutual feelings, attitudes and ways of expressing them in the patient-specialist relationship (Gelso and Hayes, 1998). It consists of several aspects that are inherent and closely intertwined with each other. These three aspects are:

- the working alliance, often considered a fundamental factor in the psychological assistance process. According to the concept of Bordin (1979, 1994 after: (Gelso and Hayes, 1998), the strength of the working alliance depends on how the patient and the therapist are) experience a mutual emotional bond – that is, the element that is the main topic of this book.
- transference – countertransference, especially emphasized in dynamic paradigms. Broadly speaking, transference is understood as the patient's perceptions of a specialist as derived from their past experience, while countertransference is the specialist's responses to the patient's transfer.
- a real relationship between the specialist and the patient – the aspect that is the most difficult to define, although intuitively quite easy to understand, involving some kind of authentic being with one another.

It is difficult to imagine a situation in which the patient could freely talk about his problems, including experienced traumas, marital or sexual problems;

DOI: 10.4324/9781003221043-6

about symptoms (depression, anxiety or eating disorders), without first establishing a relationship, gaining initial trust and bonding or experience of empathy while convinced that disclosing these matters to a specialist makes sense. Similarly, in group psychological support, including training groups, support groups or group psychotherapy, relational factors are very important – group cohesion, which is the equivalent of a therapeutic relationship in individual psychotherapy, group climate, interpersonal learning or other factors known from literature (Yalom and Leszcz, 2020). Research shows that these interpersonal elements are predictors of the effectiveness of psychotherapy. Contemporary neuroscience try to explain these issues by referring to mirror networks (Glucksman, 2020; Iacoboni, 2008; Schermer, 2010), synchronization of the cerebral hemispheres or synchronization of physiological reactions between participants of interactions (e.g. psychotherapy), which are described in this book. The above-mentioned definition and research have shown that the relationship between the patient and the professional also includes aspects of the relationship – the pattern/style of the client's relationship, the pattern/style of the therapist's bond, and the newly formed bond in the current contact, which becomes an important component of the diagnostic or therapeutic relationship, and in some cases it becomes the basic factor of change (Fonagy and Allison, 2014). Previous studies, however, assumed direct contact between the psychologist and the patient, taking into account subliminal stimuli, a wide range of non-verbal communication and sharing circumstances (being in the same room). We know little about the specifics of building such a diagnostic or therapeutic relationship in the context of modern technologies. Two main formulas of such processes should be taken into account:

- an attempt to recreate the traditional model of diagnosis and psychological assistance, using remote communication – telephone, videoconferencing programs, chats, etc.,
- the use of advanced technology (e.g. VR or mobile applications), which itself becomes the main actor and in many cases will make a diagnosis or help without the involvement of a professional psychologist.

Below we will try to consider the advantages and limitations of each of these approaches.

The traditional method of psychological diagnosis using remote communication

Originally, the use of computers in the psychologist's practice was limited mainly to the automatic evaluation of tests and questionnaires, the creation of reports and the automatic preparation of short, standardized diagnostic conclusions. In recent years, this application has significantly expanded to online testing platforms, some of which are electronic versions of traditional tools, while others are specially designed systems for electronic diagnosis, using various computer capabilities and modern software for collecting and processing diagnostic data (American Psychological Association APA Task Force on Psychological Assessment and Evaluation Guidelines, 2020). New remote communication software (e.g. Skype, Zoom, WhatsApp) has also spread, which significantly increased the possibility of distance contact between the specialist and the patient in a simple and quick way, including the use of video and several other useful options. However, is there a place for a similar therapeutic relationship and bond in such remote communication as is the case with f2f contact? In remote contact, is the therapeutic relationship and bond still an indispensable basis for professional diagnostic and therapeutic procedures?

For modern psychologists and psychotherapists it is obvious that the pattern/style of patients' attachment will be manifested in the diagnostic and therapeutic relationship, and will also be a predictor of the effectiveness of psychological interactions (Duquette, 2010; Levy et al., 2018; Mallinckrodt, 2010). At the same time, it is known from research that very often the bond formed with the psychologist is not the same as the global style of the patient's relationship (Mikulincer et al., 2013). For example, it was found that, on the one hand, the patient's safe bond was associated with a stronger therapeutic alliance in the relationship with a specialist, but on the other hand, it has been shown that preoccupied individuals form a similar form to patients with secure attachment. According to theoretical predictions, patients with avoidant individuals form a weaker therapeutic alliance with the therapist. A study by Woodhouse et al., (2003) showed that safe and preoccupied patient attachment was strongly associated with positive and negative transference. So, at least superficially, it seems that patients with secure and preoccupied individuals form a very similar type of therapeutic and transference relationship. Probably such a relationship and transference differ in the detailed dynamics known to clinicians and elusive so far in research, i.e. a patient with secure attachment feels more comfortable with expressing various emotions without fear of abandonment, while the patient will be absorbed in a known way forced internally to intensify emotions in relationship (Slade, 2016). In general – patients with avoiding attachment are less prone to reveal themselves, develop transference, in a situation of too fast and intensive building of closeness in the therapeutic relationship, they will have a tendency to drop out of therapy. At the same time, where psychological assistance oscillates around task-oriented, focus on a technically understood goal – such patients will be more involved (Janzen et al., 2008).

Attention should be paid to the aspects of the bond that lie on the therapist's side. Firstly, the therapist as a person also presents some attachment style, and secondly, the therapist within his therapeutic tasks is to facilitate and promote the formation of therapeutic bonds and relationships. Considering the fact that most patients, as mentioned above, will exhibit an insecure attachment style, this task will not be easy for the therapist, and thus the therapist's attachment style and related bonding ability will be very important. It is easy to predict that a therapist who will be able to create a secure base for his patients and be able to better withstand the emotional arousal brought in by the patient during meetings, will support change and development more. Classic studies by Mary Dozier (Dozier et al., 1994) showed that the therapist's secure attachment was a predictor of flexible response to patients' hidden needs and support for their autonomy, regardless of the patient's bonding style. On the other hand, therapists with an insecure bond were more likely to respond in a non-therapeutic manner and were prone to distract from important aspects brought in by patients. Similar results were obtained in many other studies (Daniel, 2006; Mikulincer et al., 2013; Petrowski et al., 2011; Romano et al., 2009; Tyrrell et al., 1999).The authors of the book "Attachment in grup psychotherapy" (Marmarosh et al., 2013) similarly predict the behavior of specialists in the process of group psychological help, depending on their bond style, and so:

- a therapist with a safe bond style will better tolerate stress and tension in the group, it will promote the development of mentalization in patients, it will better recognize the needs of patients with insecure attachment style, and it will be of particular importance to patients with disorganized bonds due to the instability and changeability of internal states and affect;
- on the other hand, a therapist with a preoccupied individual style may be more likely to focus on being liked and accepted by patients, he will more often detect non-verbal trauma signals, and at the same time he will be overwhelmed, he will want to save patients or he will feel no hope, it will be easier for him to promote group cohesion because he is sensitive to exclusion and a sense of community, he will better support a good therapeutic alliance, while avoiding confrontation and thus therapeutic progress;
- finally, a specialist with an avoidant style of attachment will avoid emotions and will be less empathetic, which will inhibit the emotional development of patients, will have a negative impact on patients with a preoccupied and disorganized style who will be seek emotional closeness.

All the above research reports and clinical experience come from the traditionally understood process of diagnosis and therapy, i.e. the f2f taking place. So far, relatively little is known about the therapeutic relationship when the contact with the patient takes place remotely, i.e. by phone, video-conference program or in writing.

Most psychologists are not trained to conduct diagnosis or remote therapy, because they were usually trained to the traditional form of f2f interactions, and then they carried out this form of work. Although remote forms of work have been known for a long time, a minority of specialists used them, and if they did so – only in special situations. It was only the beginning of the Covid-19 pandemic that the massive shift began – and psychologists and patients have been put in a position to either continue online or not at all. A survey by the American Psychological Association (American Psychological Association, 2020) showed three-quarters (76%) of clinicians are now solely providing remote services, primarily via phone, a designated telehealth platform or through videoconferencing software and further 16% say they are also offering remote services in addition to seeing some patients in person.

Perhaps it is for these reasons (lack of training and experience in providing on-line help) that psychologists and therapists feel exhausted when conducting online help, usually also assessing it as a worse and secondary form of working with the patient. Meanwhile, there are reports that online psychotherapy via video is better received by patients than by clinicians (Cataldo et al., 2021). Patients find remote sessions via video communicator useful, while psychologists perceive technology as an element limiting therapeutic processes. Rees and Stone (Rees and Stone, 2005) report that psychologists believe that remote consultations are inferior to f2f consultations in the field of effective building of a therapeutic alliance. Thus, there are clear differences in the perception and assessment of remote support by the specialists themselves and their patients. We will look at this in the following paragraphs.

For example, Cataldo et al., (Cataldo et al., 2021) reviewed research on psychological support provided via the Internet in the context of creating a therapeutic relationship. They also concluded that patients and psychologists assessed differently as to the possibility of creating bonds in remote contact. The research, of course, is not completely unambiguous, but the picture is that patients are generally more likely to positively assess the possibility of creating an alliance with a psychologist, and according to them, technology could serve to strengthen interaction, attention and intimacy. On the other hand, psychologists are less satisfied with remote interaction, they are full of fears and skepticism about building a therapeutic relationship of the same quality as f2f.

The role of devices, e.g. a computer, in building relationships may be important in this respect. Upon more careful consideration, it can be concluded that these devices are not only a simple medium for transmitting information, but also play a role in building the relationship between the psychologist and the patient. Some studies show that building trust in a therapeutic relationship can be influenced by a relatively faithful spatial reconstruction – that is, in a traditional contact, the psychologist and the patient share the same space in the office. This is not the case in remote assistance, so the authors of the review argue that computer mediation requires meta-communication and meta-understanding on the part of the psychologist. In other words – due to the lack of sufficient clues that are perceived naturally in the f2f process, the psychologist must perform additional mental operations that will allow him to create an image of the patient and his behavior. One of the reasons for the difficulty in performing such operations may be the lack of training and experience in remote psychological support. Thus, these operations require additional effort and energy in order to change the training acquired over the years in the traditionally conducted process of psychological assistance.

The issue of embodied, which has been described in recent years as an important part of the helping process, the sensorimotor basis of the relationship between the psychologist and the patient, may have a direct relationship with the issue described above. In this regard, important aspects will be such elements as: the physical presence of contact participants, shared external space, e.g. an office in which they spend time together, perceived smells and a whole range of subliminal stimuli (García et al., 2022; Shaw, 2004; Siegel, 2019). In online psychological contact, these aspects are much less accessible, the vision of interlocutors' bodies is limited, and the physical space around it is completely different. Some studies show that technology in the process of interacting and getting to know others is more than just a communication channel, but rather an active moderator – i.e. it creates additional meanings, distorts messages, gives messages a new meaning (Håland and Melby, 2015). Probably, mediated communication can harm emotional and other forms of relevant information, but importantly – it can also support new ways of communication and interaction (Furukawa and Driessnack, 2013; Newman et al., 2011).

This is interesting because the studies conducted so far indicate that online psychotherapy is in many cases similarly effective to f2f, and the quality of the therapeutic relationship is also similar, although some studies have shown that it builds up more slowly (Koole and Tschacher, 2016; Rees and Stone, 2005). So, as if this suggested impoverishment was not happening. García et al., (2022) argue that we should change the attitude to modern technology as an impoverished transmitter, towards becoming interested in the possibilities it offers and searching for new forms of embodied interaction. Weinberg (Weinberg, 2019, 2020) points to two aspects of online contact with the use of video. Firstly, the whole body of the interlocutor is not visible, which has its limitations, but on the other hand, the face is generally more visible, in such closeness that in real interactions is available only in close and intimate relationships. This creates new circumstances in which the psychologist must learn to read the facial expressions and deal with the limitations of the lack of other indications. One of the possibilities of such coping is the constant presence of the subject of the body in psychological contact. In other words, a psychologist or therapist can regularly ask the patient about his feelings about the body, he is sitting in some way, about the entire sensorimotor sphere, how he perceives the psychologist. It should also be taken into account that the patient also sees the face of the psychologist from a very close distance, reads (or distorts) mimic reactions much more than in direct contact. The strength of these mimic markers can lead to increased levels of anxiety and sometimes even horror in some patients, especially those who have experienced closeness traumas. Weinberg (Weinberg, 2019, 2020) also suggests that during therapeutic contact, both the patient and the psychologist turn off self-view in video communicators, usually turned on by default. Observing yourself on the screen takes a large part of the attention, makes it difficult to focus on the conversation, disrupts the entire interaction process, and strongly modifies the pro-prooceptive attention. It may also interfere with the processes between the body feeling and the body's representation in the mind, as well as the processes of bodily synchronization that are natural in live contact, i.e. that the participants of the interaction, entering into a deeper relationship, unconsciously imitate their body postures, and there is also an automatic synchronization at the physiological level.

The next two important aspects to consider are technological awareness and ethical and legal issues. Awareness of technological progress and its impact on diagnostic and therapeutic processes is an important issue and task for a psychologist. The psychologist should be familiar with the whole range of modern diagnostic and therapeutic techniques, which gives the opportunity to expand the existing range of professional opportunities. This is important because in the case of the inability to meet the f2f patient, the use of some equivalent of a diagnostic task may be of key importance. Also important is the knowledge of psychometric or predictive properties in clinical diagnosis and the possibility of the formation of diagnostic artifacts related to the specifics of distance contact (American Psychological Association APA Task Force on Psychological Assessment and Evaluation Guidelines, 2020). It is also important in this situation that the psychologist is able to efficiently use the programs and equipment he uses, as well as he can efficiently use analog tools (e.g. tests with blocks, puzzles, toys, other props). The same efficiency in the use of devices and programs should also be achieved by the patient, and it is not so obvious, especially in the elderly population (Czaja et al., 2019). A very important task in this respect will be the psychologist's instruction in the initial phase of contact in order to be able to move on to the substantive aspects later. These issues are not only important in technical terms, but also as an important element in building relationships and bonds between the psychologist and the patient – if they are both preoccupied with technical matters, it will be difficult to get down to relational aspects, emotions and bond building (Rosen et al., 2016).

When it comes to ethical and legal issues, we will highlight two important issues here. The first is about keeping records and collecting data using electronic tools. It is important for the psychologist and the institution in which he works to comply with the highest standards of securing data obtained during diagnosis and therapy. The second issue concerns the use of videoconferencing programs that provide encryption and prevent eavesdropping on conversations during the meeting. Although these are extremely important issues, their detailed discussion goes beyond the thematic framework of the book and we refer readers to the principles (American Psychological Association APA Task Force on Psychological Assessment and Evaluation Guidelines, 2020), ethical and legal codes in individual countries. In addition, you can see the study prepared by APA and AGPA – American Group Psychotherapy Association on the recommendation of programs for remote psychological assistance https://www.agpa.org/home/practice-resources/connecting-online.

In the context of this book, it should be mentioned that these issues, accepted as if automatically in psychological help provided to f2f, are not so obvious in online contact. when the patient comes to the psychologist's office, he personally automatically assumes that the help will be provided in accordance with the law, the data about him will be protected and the psychologist will ensure the comfort of confidentiality – they are the default, basic and necessary condition for the patient's sense of security, which is the starting point for further creation relationship with a specialist. These issues are not so obvious in online contact and should be the subject of reflection for a psychologist and an important task when deciding to provide online services. In this respect, it will also be important to sensitize the patient to aspects lying on his side – for example, where the patient connects from, whether he or she has the comfort of talking freely about all matters, whether there are additional disruptive stimuli such as noise or other multimedia included. which will influence the patient's attention and thus also the effectiveness of diagnosis and building a therapeutic bond.

Transition from face to face contact to remote relationship

Basic concepts and phenomena, e.g. behaviors, boundaries, goals and therapeutic contract, must be modified to the new situation in which there is no direct contact, and both parties must cooperate even more closely in creating the space of the therapeutic relationship (Mazri and Fiorentini, 2017). For example, consider a situation over which the therapist has no control, namely, that during a session, the connection on the telephone or internet line is lost. Maintaining the continuity of such a meeting is somewhat of a hassle and should be found in the online therapy preliminary arrangements. It may happen that the patient, in an unexpected and sometimes even very difficult moment of the session, will be left alone with himself, so the contract should include an agreement on the procedure in such a case, e.g. using other communication channels (e.g. after a while connecting phone calls) and the patient's behavior at that moment – for example, that he should use these breaks as an opportunity to deepen his reflection on himself. These findings are also important because there may be times when they will come across various difficult experiences of the patient in the past, for example, during such a breakdown, they will re-experience a type of rejection or abandonment (Weinberg and Rolnick, 2019b).

Another issue that definitely distinguishes the psychological contact of f2f from remote is the issue of self-presence. In online contact, setting the camera is seemingly a small technical matter, but in fact it is extremely important in the context of creating a therapeutic relationship. Previous studies have shown that an extremely important part of the feeling of presence between the patient and the therapist is creating an almost illusion that the person is really present with us (Lombard and Ditton, 1997; Russell, 2015). On the other hand, positioning the face too closely on the screen may give a feeling of too much intimacy and the patient may over-read or distort the facial expressions that are the basis for reading emotions. Wenberg and Rolnick refer to Porges (Porges, 2011), who, in his polyvagal theory, emphasizes the key issue of the face in interpersonal communication and who indicates that people regulate each other based on facial expressions and tone of voice. In this case, one of the unique characteristics of online therapy is that the specialist and the patient see each other's faces much more clearly than in the actual f2f relationship. At the same time, the psychologist must remember not to neglect the rest of the body, from which we can get a lot of information about the emotional state of the other side, you can find in his body language (Aviezer et al., 2012). We wrote a few paragraphs earlier about the issues of embodied communication and the body in online therapy.

An important element is also the ability to make and maintain eye contact through a video communicator, which is to give a special sense of awareness. It is very easy to get interested in some objects in the environment in a remote contact, which are different from the objects in the patient's environment. A special element here is the issue of distractors from a device, e.g. a telephone or a computer – e.g. notifications about incoming messages may be displayed, information or advertisements may appear when the browser window is open. These elements should be controlled as much as possible, and these issues should be agreed with the patient, so that during online meetings he should also be mindful of contact with the specialist.

It is also worth realizing that the psychologist appears in the patient's private space, which has various consequences. The psychologist is on the computer screen in front of which the patient probably spends a lot of time working, running errands or relaxing. For many people, this is a natural environment, and the device may in some ways be treated unconsciously as an extension of the body or self – which will in some way facilitate contact and accelerate the formation of a therapeutic relationship and continuity between sessions. At the same time, appearing in the patient's private space may be uncomfortable, and at the initial stage the patient may not be aware of it. For example, when applying for therapy for reasons that the patient associates with work, he may not have any reluctance to talk about relations at work in the apartment. However, when, as a result of deepening the understanding of his problems, he may no longer be able to speak openly and loudly about relationships with household members – even with the door closed. At the initiative of the psychologist, these issues must be included in the initial contracting process.

There is also the question of the technical skills of using a computer, programs or other devices for remote communication, both by the patient and the psychologist. This gives a special dimension to the relationship through forced cooperation on technical aspects, e.g. determining whether they can hear each other well, see well, or something stutters, suggest ways to increase the comfort of work.

Some aspects that distinguish f2f from remote contact have been described above and it should be emphasized that these are not all aspects. Below, after Wainberg (Weinberg and Rolnick, 2019a), we present some basic principles that are important for a specialist in building a contract and therapeutic relationship with the patient. So, the following recommendations should be considered:

- It is good to combine online and f2f meetings, and in particular to emphasize the possibility of face-to-face meetings before moving on to regular online contact. If f2f contact is not possible now, schedule it with the patient as soon as possible;
- Plan the frequency of online meetings as if you were doing it in stationary contact. Typically, online therapy results in fewer missed sessions, which has also been confirmed by studies. At the same time, during the planned leaves of the therapist/patient, one should not make an appointment, although it would be technically possible;
- Make the patient aware of the issue of the distance from the computer screen during the online meeting – it is best to discuss the needs and comfort in this respect with the patient and make the patient sensitive to specific situations, so that he can inform about his perception of closeness or distance with the therapist. Also note that in some computers the camera may be placed in a different place than the center of the screen at eye level, which may cause distortions, as the therapist's or patient's eyesight will be directed in a different direction – then you should consider installing an external camera;
- The psychologist or therapist should be strongly focused on the patient, which we also wrote about earlier. Keep distractions to a minimum, and if you do and you still have a problem with concentration, consider this in terms of countertransference;
- Ask the patient for help in controlling the surroundings. In f2f meetings, the psychologist has control over the environment (office), and during online meetings, he loses this control. Agree with the patient to meet from a quiet room, preferably from the same place each time where they can feel and speak freely. Set rules so that meetings are not held while driving or lying out of bed. Prepare the patient and conduct psychoeducation in this regard. Some things that are obvious to a specialist are not like that to the patient;
- Technological aspects are also an important part – it is best, if possible, that the patient should not use a phone or tablet, but rather connect to a computer that provides a stable large image (all the more important in group therapy where there are many people on the screen). Explain to patients the issue of a large stable image, discuss with the patient the issue

of internet speed and the use of headphones for better comfort and no feedback. The psychologist or therapist can provide written technical instructions on the specific technology they use, such as how to operate the Zoom program or how to set up useful functions in it. It is good when a psychologist efficiently uses technology at a basic level, at the same time he does not have to be an expert in these matters. It may often happen that a patient will be able to instruct a psychologist on how to solve technological problems – do not rule out such an option and be prepared for such dynamics;

- Consider writing a written contract for all online therapy arrangements;
- Discuss with the patient the emergency intervention procedure, which is especially important for patients with fragile egos and primitive defense mechanisms who are exposed to emotional crises, impulses or suicide attempts, e.g. with borderline personality disorder. Check emergency telephone numbers with the patient, consider giving the patient the name and telephone number of an emergency contact, or their doctor. Establish a crisis management procedure (e.g. for the patient to call the nearest hospital or ask someone for help);
- Remember not to ignore any situations that happen on the screen and in the patient's environment during the meeting. In f2f therapy, incidents that take place in the therapy room are commented on and analyzed – why should it be different during online therapy;
- Establish a procedure with the patient in the event of a connection failure, e.g. contact by phone, so that the session can be continued relatively effectively and the patient knows what to do in case of such unforeseen situations;
- Consultations and therapy via the Internet can take place with patients from all over the world – be sure to set the hours taking into account time zones. Also remember about cultural differences, be sensitive to them, explore the norms of this culture;
- It would be good for both the patient and the specialist to turn off the view of themselves – "self view" enabled by default in most videoconference programs, so that people see themselves from the side of the screen like in a mirror. Seeing oneself increases self-awareness, but at the same time takes away a lot of attention that should be devoted to the patient, and also distracts from the therapeutic relationship. Therefore, it is advisable that both the patient and the psychologist (or participants of the therapeutic group turn off the "self view" function;
- It is good for the psychologist to show his vitality, not to sit still, but to change his position, nodding his head, gesturing with his hands, etc. This will show the patient interest and stimulate the dynamics of contact;
- Check and comply with legal, ethical and data protection issues. It may be different in different countries;

- A psychologist, even if he conducts meetings from home, should dress officially, as he would be dressed in the institution where he conducts consultations or f2f therapies. If a patient is dressed atypically, it should be included as standard in the analysis during a diagnostic or therapeutic session.

Modern technologies as the main element of psychological diagnosis and therapy

In the previous section, we focused on diagnosis and psychological therapy understood in a traditional way, in which there is a therapeutic relationship and a bond between the clinician and the patient – only mediated by remote communication devices. What about diagnosis and therapy, where the specialist as a person is completely or almost completely replaced by modern technologies?

More and more data indicate that the use of modern technologies can be useful in the prevention, diagnosis and improvement of mental health, it can improve mental health, such as anxiety and depression, in various patient populations (Campbell et al., 2014a, 2014b; Lattie et al., 2019a, 2019b). At the same time, it should be noted that there are serious limitations in many areas, including: currently limited scientific evidence for some interventions, the lack of technical and medical standards for mobile mental health applications, and unresolved ethical and legal issues, such as privacy protection (Ienca et al., 2018; Mohr et al., 2017; Wexler and Reiner, 2019). There is also a lack of data on the formation of a therapeutic relationship and bond – an important aspect related to the effectiveness of an intervention. These data are also missing because, going beyond the traditional paradigm of the clinician-human and patient-human meeting, there is a lack of an appropriate vision, methodology and understanding of the relationship between the patient and the application, program or device. By reviewing selected methods below: virtual reality, mobile applications and computer games, we will devote a few reflections to the above-mentioned issues.

Virtual reality VR in diagnosis and psychological therapy

What may speak in favor of modern technologies in relation to, for example, traditional psychological diagnosis, are the limitations of this traditional diagnosis. For example, self-report tools are based on declarations, thinking about hypothetical situations, describe the general behavior of the respondent, and are devoid of a specific life context. Some patients with limited cognitive abilities, under stress or with psychiatric symptoms may show poor understanding of items. In contact with a psychologist, patients, especially those with low self-esteem or other personality constructions, may show a particular susceptibility to social approval, and in the case of children, only parents can evaluate emotions, behavior and getting to know their children. The above aspects selectively show the limitations of traditional diagnosis, which therefore often shows low accuracy (Duckworth and Yeager, 2015; Simmering et al., 2019). The question of context may be particularly important in this respect – behaviors may or may not occur in various contexts (e.g. persistence in pursuing a hobby vs perseverance in school), and real behavior usually differs from hypothetically considered and declared in psychological questionnaires (Bostyn et al., 2018; Simmering et al., 2019). In this case, virtual reality can prove to be an extremely useful tool for psychological assessment.

Virtual reality is an artificial 3D environment capable of reproducing reality and its accompanying experiences, in which people can also interact as if it were happening in reality. VR provides almost complete immersion in this experience stimulating a higher level of active involvement. According to some, VR is an appropriate, and maybe even better tool for assessing behavior in psychology, giving the possibility of observing the patient in various aspects and contexts, for example when assessing risky behavior in a work situation. VR is able to map the real-world attitude to risk – without exposing people to real risk, embodied learning to assess and defend against risk, and real-time physiological measurement (de-Juan-Ripoll et al., 2018).

VR is already used in the field of psychological help and psychotherapy, and the research on this tool to date is promising. In the treatment of anxiety disorders in the CBT paradigm, both based on virtual reality exposure therapy and on more complex interventions, the method using VR obtained similar results to the traditionally conducted CBT therapy (Carl et al., 2019; Eichenberg and Wolters, 2012; Valmaggia et al., 2016). Very promising results have also been obtained in the treatment of psychotic patients – social skills training, training to develop the theory of mind, social cognition and re-cognition of emotions have shown good effectiveness (Freeman et al., 2019; Nijman et al., 2019; Pot-Kolder et al., 2018; Rus-Calafell et al., 2018). Very interesting interventions have been formulated for productive symptoms, where patients can talk to an avatar that matches the voices heard as hallucinations, and then these patients can control such an avatar (Craig et al., 2018; Leff et al., 2013). VR has also shown usefulness in the treatment of eating disorders, addiction to psychoactive substances (Clus et al., 2018; Kim and Lee, 2019; Liu et al., 2020; Pericot-Valverde et al., 2019) and mood disorder (Clus et al., 2018; Kim and Lee, 2019), although some results were inconclusive, and others indicated that VR could be a complementary technique to standard methods.

Working with patients using VR can lead to a situation of automated treatment, and such attempts have already been made. Of course, this has its advantages related to the availability of treatment, where you will be able to get help quickly, without waiting in line for the availability of a specialist. Moreover, it may be useful in intensifying or supplementing standard treatment, e.g. homework between f2f sessions or as maintenance therapy after completion of therapy with a therapist. Of course, this also carries some dangers. If such automated forms of therapy become widespread, it may be a situation of self-medication without prior professional psychological diagnosis, unforeseen side effects or deterioration during therapy. The second element concerns the most important thing in this book – that is, the therapeutic re-lationship and the bond with the patient. Two scenarios can be envisioned here. In the first VR, we treat it as one of the techniques, but the entire diagnostic and therapeutic process takes place with the participation of a psychologist, where all other elements of the psychologist-patient contact are preserved. In the second, therapeutic VR technology is available for purchase in generally accessible stores or via the Internet, and patients themselves, and even other third parties (e.g. parents to their children), serve the therapy without the control of a professional.

There is also a possibility that in some cases a therapeutic relationship or a bond between the specialist and the patient is not needed (?) As evidenced by research using platforms with self-help programs, where patients in some cases get quite good results using educational materials and scheduled tasks in an automated computer program.

Applications for mobile phones, tablets and computers

Another modern approach to diagnosis, prevention and psychological therapy is telephone applications. There are many applications related to mental health, and with the dynamically changing situation on the market of this type of software, it is difficult to determine their number. According to some reports, there are probably more than 10.000 such applications currently available (Torous et al., 2018). It should be noted right away that many of these ap-plications do not have strong evidence of their effectiveness confirmed by research, which is a certain difficulty both for the users themselves and for clinicians who want to recommend something to their patients. Quite often, the choices are made on the basis of the assessments and reviews of the users themselves, which appear in mobile online stores with such applications, which according to scientific criteria is not a sufficient proof of credibility, safety and effectiveness, and vice versa – can also give unreliable results (Huang and Bashir, 2017; Marshall et al., 2019a).

The content contained in the applications most often includes some kind of self-assessment (self-diagnosis) carried out by the user, providing psychoedu-cational materials and various types of exercises, most often borrowed from cognitive-behavioral therapy. One can envision the broad benefits of mental health enhancement applications, similar to those presented in the entire field of online psychological support, e.g. accessibility for people with low socio-economic status, better access for people from smaller localities, where treatment options may be limited, anonymity of help, and therefore reduced possibility of stigmatization and self-stigmatization of patients, naturalness of help due to the fact that most people are smartphone users anyway. Especially for children and adolescents, it can be a natural, attractive and simply preferable form of receiving mental health information (Bowers et al., 2013; Jones et al., 2014; Sakai et al., 2014; Wang et al., 2018).

Already carried research have shown that mental health applications can be effective in reducing anxiety and depression. Effect sizes in these studies have been estimated to be low to moderate. At the same time, it should be added that these studies have significant methodological limitations and show diversity that does not allow direct comparisons of individual studies, e.g. differences in the duration of the intervention, the intensity of application use and the lack of data from longer observations (Firth et al., 2017; Firth et al., 2017; Fleming et al., 2018; Howells et al., 2016).

One RCT study by (Bakker et al., 2018a) compared patients using three applications: MoodMission, MoodPrism and MoodKit, with a 30-day waiting list control. Users of all three applications experienced an improvement in mental well-being, and those using MoodMission and MoodKit experienced a decrease in depression. The analyzes revealed that the change was mediated by an increase in coping self-efficacy, i.e. individual's ability to comprehend their own emotions. Despite the recognition of the effectiveness based on declarations in these studies, the effects in the real world were not assessed.

Just MoodMission is one of the best-known mental health improvement apps. The website of the developers of the application is available at https://moodmission.com/, and the application itself is available for download in stores offering applications for both Android and Ios smartphones. It is an application that uses CBT strategies for users (patients) reporting anxiety and depressed mood. Bakker et al., (2018b) write that MoodMission was created with the intention of users learning how to use strategies themselves to reduce depressed mood and anxiety, especially at low, subclinical intensity and also as an addition to psychotherapy. Users estimate their mood, which is some kind of self-diagnosis, and then the software provides a list of five CBT-based tasks which have been called "Missions". Using the application is focused on the ability to cope with stressors and increase emotional self-awareness and coping self-efficacy, i.e. individual's ability to comprehend their own emotions, leading to positive mental health outcomes (O'Toole et al., 2014). The missions are designed in a simple way so that they can be performed independently by the users. Each step can be completed in 5–10 minutes. The application has been designed for a wide audience and uses intelligent algorithms to adjust tasks based on the previous self-diagnosis and individual preferences.

In one of the systematic reviews of research on various applications for people with anxiety and depression (Marshall et al., 2019b), the authors checked what percentage of the creators of these applications:

- declare the effectiveness of their application confirmed by scientific research;

- involve mental health experts in the app development process;
- collaborate with a research institution, medical institution or other institutions;
- offers the application free of charge.

The results showed that for 3.41% of the applications, studies were conducted to justify their effectiveness, with most of these studies being undertaken directly by the developers of the applications themselves. 30.38% of app developers said they collaborated with experts; 20.48% had connections with a state body, scientific institution or medical institution; and 74.06% were free. The authors conclude that future work must include a specific methodology that will facilitate the proper conduct of more research and greater input from mental health experts in the development of these applications.

Another, puzzling issue is the issue of building a therapeutic relationship and bond, because in this case with whom to build it? Can there be a relationship with a smartphone, tablet, application, or maybe with an imaginary therapist imagined by the patient using such an application?

It turns out that this topic has been discussed in the literature, and the conclusion is that people, especially when human attachment figures are less accessible, tend to become attached to objects other than people (Hooley and Wilson-Murphy, 2012; Keefer et al., 2012). This is similar to the well-known concept of transitional objects described by (Winnicott, 1953). Research has shown that young people are more likely to develop a bond with the phone and experience discomfort when it is not available, and the bonding style of individual people is related to the way they use the objects to which they become attached. For example, subjects with a higher level of attachment anxiety tended to seek contact with the phone (Konok et al., 2016). The results of these studies are ambiguous – it is not known whether the respondents were looking for the telephone itself – the object, or the interpersonal contacts that can be made via the telephone. Other studies have shown that well-functioning people can benefit from attachment to various kinds of objects: possession of these objects can be soothing in times of stress, can help regulate emotions, can increase life satisfaction and even be associated with better mental health (Myers, 1985; Sherman, 2019; Wapner et al., 1990; Wiseman and Watt, 2004). However, many unanswered questions arise. For example, better well-being may occur due to the strengthening of the defense mechanism of avoidance, or in today's consumptive times of self-satisfaction as the owner of a valuable item. Moreover, it might turn out that the object itself, e.g. a telephone, may somehow be associated with real people – for example, a young person received a telephone call from his parents as a gift. It should also be distinguished that the very use of the telephone as such is another thing, and the use of applications intended to improve mental health. These are because they offer substantive content and interventions that serve this very purpose.

It should also be noted that the above studies did not deal directly with the therapeutic relationship and bond. The authors of a recent review (Henson et al., 2019) on the therapeutic Alliance in the context of mobile applications for mental health express their surprise at such a low percentage of research in this area, given the number and use of such applications. They identified 5 studies in this area, and in no case was the evaluation of the therapeutic alliance the primary goal. The conclusions of this review are that smartphones as an additional component of therapy can lead to increased engagement and adherence, and that the therapeutic Alliance increases the ability to communicate with the clinician beyond standard therapy meetings. It is unclear, however, how the therapeutic relationship can change with varying degrees of clinician involvement and when interventions are performed only using a smartphone. Currently, mobile applications mainly try to translate cognitive-behavioral therapy textbooks into smartphone formats, but at the same time have brought less benefits than expected. Perhaps the issue of a therapeutic relationship, attachment or working Alliance could explain this phenomenon. So in this regard, we have more unknowns than known, and the above sentences are purely speculative and rather outline areas for further research.

Video games in the process of diagnosis and therapy

According to 2019 data for the computer and video game industry in America, 65% of adults play video games, 75% have at least one player in their household, 54% of gamers are men, 79% of gamers believe that the game provides mentally stimulated, 78% of players declare a sense of relaxation and relaxation while playing, and 74% of parents believe that gaming can have an educational value for their (Vajawat et al., 2021).

Serious games or Applied games, or games whose creation from the very beginning is directed towards goals other than just entertainment, have recently gained great popularity in the field of psychology and psychiatry. Based on the principles of gamification, they target psychosocial and cognitive domains in line with deficits in various mental disorders. They have already been used for cognitive behavioral therapy, cognitive training and rehabilitation, behavior modification, social motivation, attention enhancement, and biological feedback. Research shows their usefulness in ADHD, autism spectrum disorders, eating disorders, post-traumatic stress disorder, impulse control disorders, depression, schizophrenia, dementia, and even in the process of healthy aging. At the same time, it should be remembered that this method, due to insufficient scientific data, still remains experimental. Either way, the combination of mental health and gaming seems to be very promising, with benefits over the course of other remote methods, as described above (Aboujaoude et al., 2015).

People who play video games may interact with virtual worlds, but that doesn't make the experience any less real for gamers. The emotions and states that people may experience while playing the game can have therapeutic implications in the hands of a qualified and prepared therapist. Thanks to knowledge about games or just curiosity in this area, it is possible to establish contact with patients, in particular with children and adolescents, because games can provide a good platform for understanding, where it is difficult to find other topics in the initial contact.

As for the diagnostic part, games can quite often be used as a projection method. A conversation about what games the patient plays, what characters he or she impersonates, what he wants to achieve with them, can tell a lot about his attitudes, emotions and needs. Franco reports (Franco, 2016) that according to the Entertainment Software Association, the most players – 31% – played social games, which indicates that players can reach for them to meet social needs. On the other hand, action games and horror films can provide patients with a new perspective on themselves, because by meeting their pleasure while watching or using violence, users can gain insight into these instinctive spheres of their own psyche (Krzywinska, 2015).

An exemplary product in this area would be Akili Interactive Labs, Boston, MA, USA, the trade name of which is EndeavorRx. In 2020, the US Food and Drug Administration (FDA) included EndeavorRx on its list as a therapy for children with ADHD.

It is a game for computers, telephones and tablets, which belongs to the so-called "serious game" or "applied game", that is, as already mentioned, from the very beginning its creation was focused on goals other than entertainment. The game was developed for kids to improve attention control, more specifically to manage competing tasks and to efficiently (flexibly) shift attention between tasks. The game uses an original and proprietary algorithm that personalizes the game difficulty level for each player.

Considering the purpose of the game, it will be useful especially for children with ADHD syndrome, and evidence of its effectiveness is confirmed by research published in The Lancet Digital Health (Kollins et al., 2020). The game is based on gamification, which increases the motivation of users, presents modern graphics, which increases its attractiveness, includes a reward loop and uses adaptation mechanisms in real time – the game level adjusts in real time to the detected current user level.

The mechanism of the game was created in such a way that the challenges faced by a young player are attractive to him and require focus. The players do not mindlessly go through the individual stages, but are faced with all sorts of challenges encouraging them to carefully, and even repeatedly, go through individual games. Points earned in the game can be exchanged for hero skins and other rewards offered by the game, which, together with attractive graphics, creates a modern and child-attractive fun.

The main essence of the game is to steer the vehicle that moves over the track line so that it does not fall off the road, while collecting certain objects and avoiding others. There is some kind of multitasking, with a need to toggle your attention, pursue goals, and avoid others.

It is recommended that children with ADHD use the game 5 days a week for about 25 minutes, for a period of one month, and the next month of the game is to bring further results. Based on research, 68% of parents of children noticed symptomatic improvement, 73% of children showed improvement in attention function, and no undesirable side effects were noted (Kollins et al., 2020, 2021). Information about the game can also be obtained directly at https://www.endeavorrx.com/, where we will receive detailed information, references to research and the opportunity to see trailers video.

As can be seen from the above general description, relational issues in interventions involving computer games are not taken into account. Two conclusions can be drawn from this – either in this type of disorder, the issue of relationality does not play such a role, or the issue of relationality exists but has not been properly controlled (e.g. it is not known how the qualification meetings for examinations with specialists proceeded in detail, or whether the attention of the parents of the children was not in more focused on children during the research, if the parents did not accompany the child while playing).

What's next?

In recent years, more and more studies have been conducted, which can be broadly described by the category: Psychoinformatics (Markowetz et al., 2014; Yarkoni, 2012). They consist in diagnosing and predicting certain psychological variables or behaviors based on the analysis of people's activity on the Internet, in particular in social networks. A growing body of research presents empirical evidence that data from human-machine interactions (e.g. Facebook, Twitter, and Sina) can be analyzed to effectively predict psychological variables.

For example, on the basis of research on the likes of almost 60.000 Facebook users, researchers have shown the possibility of testing individual people's sexuality, ethnicity, political attitudes – and, what is particularly interesting, personalities according to the Big Five Theory. The correlation suggests that about 16% of the variance of likes on Facebook and the overlap of the personality test (Kosinski et al., 2014; Qiu et al., 2012) report that personality traits such as neuroticism and agreeableness can also be predicted based on activity on Tweeter. Other studies showed that extroverts and people with low conscientiousness used WhatsApp more often and longer (Montag et al., 2015). Users who use smartphones intensively more often distort the time they spend with the phone in their hands (Montag et al., 2015). This is shown by facts known from psychology: extroverts have more contacts with others and will contact them more often using social networks or smartphones, while people with low conscientiousness will use these media more often and longer, but for different reasons – delaying their daily life tasks or inadequately estimating the time needed to complete them.

As it was written in this chapter, modern technologies are able to assess and change various mental functions of a person, and we will probably soon use the data provided by a car to identify road behavior (impulsiveness, aggressiveness, recklessness, etc.) (Han and Yang, 2009; Imkamon et al., 2008), and other devices, such as a refrigerator connected to the Internet, which will show eating habits and help in adhering to the diet of people with various problems, eg with eating disorders (Luo et al., 2009).

We still have little knowledge about the use of modern technologies in applied psychology to merge individual data from research and clinical practice into a coherent system of diagnosis and psychological help. However, we can make predictions in this regard and prepare for some pitfalls. It is not difficult to imagine that in diagnosis and psychological assistance the traditional methods such as clinical interview or paper-and-pencil questionnaires will be replaced mostly by other data: performing a task in a smartphone application, playing a computer game, analyzing activity in social networks or experimenting with behavior. with the use of virtual reality. What will be the role of the psychologist, the therapeutic relationship, and will it be needed at all?

The first issue that will need to be resolved is the question of the equivalence of data collected by technologies with classical tests, their reliability and validity, in comparison with the hitherto measures used in psychology. We know that standard versions of psychological questionnaires performed on paper or via an online form exhibit similar psychmetric properties (Riva et al., 2003). We do not know, however, what about other data – how the participation in a computer game relates to, for example, a decision-making situation at work or giving likes on social networks with real behavior during a social gathering last weekend. The methods used in psychology to date have been far from perfect, but at the same time, over the years of experience, specialists have developed ways to deal with these imperfections, which allowed for effective help. Perhaps modern methods will prove to be more effective than the existing ones, but they will also require changes in the behavior of psychologists, learning to integrate data from various sources. If the change is gradual, possibly as a gradual evolutionary change, specialists will slowly learn and change. However, today's nature of modern technology shows rather revolutionary, that is, a rapid and sudden change, which is best shown by the outbreak of the Covid 19 pandemic and the transition of psychologists overnight to new ways of working that they have not used until now.

Secondly, a slightly less abrupt change can be imagined, and the use of modern technologies by patients in diagnosis and therapy. Conversations with a teenager about computer games, e.g. what characters he or she impersonates, what these characters think and what motives they have, can be treated as a modification of projection methods by learning about the internal structure of our patient. In addition, talking to the patient about how he reacts to behavior in social media or preferences regarding the websites visited can allow for a deeper understanding of our patients. We do not mention, of course, that talking about important areas (e.g. computer games for a teenager) will probably be an important element in building a therapeutic relationship and relationship.

Thirdly, it is possible to imagine a situation where modern technologies do a lot of work by giving us information about cognitive functions, social functioning or disorders in the patient, which in turn will save a lot of time for a standard interview, questionnaire study or behavioral experiment conducted for this purpose. pores in the psychological office. The time saved during the meeting with the patient itself will be able to be used for a conversation between two people, establishing an appropriate relationship, and even a deep bond – especially if this in further research on the interaction of psychology – modern technologies will not lose its importance.

Can the therapeutic bond and relationship lose its importance? Science today can not answer this question. It can be imagined that the whole wide diagnostic and therapeutic trend emphasizing the importance of the intervention itself (without taking into account the relationship) will completely dominate psychology and the area of mental health. Many studies show the possibility of treatment with a little specialist involvement or commitment at the stage of creating a game, application, etc., but not at the stage of treatment. As if the relationship in this case was not important.

However, on the other hand, a whole series of other studies, especially in psychodynamic and interpersonal paradigms, show the great importance of the therapeutic relationship. Perhaps this is due to some differences that are not available to science at the moment, where under certain conditions a therapeutic bond and relationship are necessary, and under different conditions, circumstances or characteristics of the patient, the very nature of the technical interventions is crucial. Knowing and resolving these issues is a clear task for the next years facing the entire field of psychology and mental health.

References

Aboujaoude, E., Salame, W., Naim, L. (2015). Telemental health: A status update. *World Psychiatry*, 14(2). 10.1002/wps.20218

American Psychological Association. (2020). *Psychologists embrace telehealth to prevent the spread of COVID-19*. Retrieved August. https://www.apaservices.org/practice/legal/technology/psychologists-embrace-telehealth

American Psychological Association APA Task Force on Psychological Assessment and Evaluation Guidelines. (2020). *APA Guidelines for Psychological Assessment and Evaluation*.

Aviezer, H., Trope, Y., Todorov, A. (2012). Body cues, not facial expressions, discriminate between intense positive and negative emotions. *Science*, 338(6111). 10.1126/science.1224313

Bakker, D., Kazantzis, N., Rickwood, D., Rickard, N. (2018a). A randomized controlled trial of three smartphone apps for enhancing public mental health. *Behaviour Research and Therapy*, 109, 75–83. 10.1016/J.BRAT.2018.08.003

Bakker, D., Kazantzis, N., Rickwood, D., Rickard, N. (2018b). Development and Pilot Evaluation of Smartphone-Delivered Cognitive Behavior Therapy Strategies for Mood- and Anxiety-Related Problems: MoodMission. *Cognitive and Behavioral Practice*, 25(4), 496–514. 10.1016/J.CBPRA.2018.07.002

Bostyn, D.H., Sevenhant, S., Roets, A. (2018). Of Mice, Men, and Trolleys: Hypothetical Judgment Versus Real-Life Behavior in Trolley-Style Moral Dilemmas. *Psychological Science*, 29(7). 10.1177/0956797617752640

Bowers, H., Manion, I., Papadopoulos, D., Gauvreau, E. (2013). Stigma in school-based mental health: Perceptions of young people and service providers. *Child and Adolescent Mental Health*, 18(3). 10.1111/j.1475-3588.2012.00673.x

Campbell, A.N.C., Nunes, E.V., Matthews, A.G., Stitzer, M., Miele, G.M., Polsky, D., Turrigiano, E., Walters, S., McClure, E.A., Kyle, T.L., Wahle, A., van Veldhuisen, P., Goldman, B., Babcock, D., Stabile, P.Q., Winhusen, T., Ghitza, U.E. (2014a). Internet-delivered treatment for substance abuse: A multisite randomized controlled trial. *American Journal of Psychiatry*, 171(6). 10.1176/appi.ajp.2014.13081055

Campbell, A.N.C., Nunes, E.V., Matthews, A.G., Stitzer, M., Miele, G.M., Polsky, D., Turrigiano, E., Walters, S., McClure, E.A., Kyle, T.L., Wahle, A., van Veldhuisen, P., Goldman, B., Babcock, D., Stabile, P.Q., Winhusen, T., Ghitza, U. E. (2014b). Internet-delivered treatment for substance abuse: A multisite randomized controlled trial. *American Journal of Psychiatry*, 171(6), 683–690. 10.1176/APPI.AJP.2014.13081055

Carl, E., Stein, A.T., Levihn-Coon, A., Pogue, J.R., Rothbaum, B., Emmelkamp, P., Asmundson, G.J.G., Carlbring, P., Powers, M.B. (2019). Virtual reality exposure therapy for anxiety and related disorders: A meta-analysis of randomized controlled trials. *Journal of Anxiety Disorders*, 61. 10.1016/j.janxdis.2018.08.003

Cataldo, F., Chang, S., Mendoza, A., Buchanan, G. (2021). A Perspective on Client-Psychologist Relationships in Videoconferencing Psychotherapy: Literature Review. *JMIR Mental Health*, 8(2). 10.2196/19004

Clus, D., Larsen, M.E., Lemey, C., Berrouiguet, S. (2018). The use of virtual reality in patients with eating disorders: Systematic review. In *Journal of Medical Internet Research*, 20(4). 10.2196/jmir.7898

Craig, T.K., Rus-Calafell, M., Ward, T., Leff, J.P., Huckvale, M., Howarth, E., Emsley, R., Garety, P.A. (2018). AVATAR therapy for auditory verbal hallucinations in people with psychosis: a single-blind, randomised controlled trial. *The Lancet Psychiatry*, 5(1). 10.1016/S2215-0366(17)30427-3

Czaja, S.J., Boot, W.R., Charness, N., Rogers, W.A. (2019). *Designing for Older Adults: Principles and Creative Human Factors Approaches* (3rd ed.). CRC Press. https://www.routledge.com/Designing-for-Older-Adults-Principles-and-Creative-Human-Factors-Approaches/Czaja-Boot-Charness-Rogers/p/book/9781138053663

Daniel, S.I.F. (2006). Adult attachment patterns and individual psychotherapy: A review. In *Clinical Psychology Review*, 26(8). 10.1016/j.cpr.2006.02.001

de-Juan-Ripoll, C., Soler-Domínguez, J.L., Guixeres, J., Contero, M., Gutiérrez, N.Á., Alcañiz, M. (2018). Virtual reality as a new approach for risk taking assessment. *Frontiers in Psychology*, 9(DEC), 2532. 10.3389/FPSYG.2018.02532/BIBTEX

Dozier, M., Cue, K.L., Barnett, L. (1994). Clinicians as Caregivers: Role of Attachment Organization in Treatment. *Journal of Consulting and Clinical Psychology*, 62(4), 793–800. 10.1037//0022-006X.62.4.793

Duckworth, A.L., Yeager, D.S. (2015). Measurement Matters: Assessing Personal Qualities Other Than Cognitive Ability for Educational Purposes. 44(4), 237–251. 10.3102/0013189X15584327

Duquette, P. (2010). Reality matters: Attachment, the real relationship, and change in psychotherapy. In *American Journal of Psychotherapy*, 64(2). 10.1176/appi.psychotherapy.2010.64.2.127

Eichenberg, C., Wolters, C. (2012). Virtual Realities in the Treatment of Mental Disorders: A Review of the Current State of Research. In *Virtual Reality in Psychological, Medical and Pedagogical Applications*. 10.5772/50094

Firth, J., Torous, J., Nicholas, J., Carney, R., Pratap, A., Rosenbaum, S., Sarris, J. (2017). The efficacy of smartphone-based mental health interventions for depressive symptoms: a meta-analysis of randomized controlled trials. *World Psychiatry*, 16(3). 10.1002/wps.20472

Firth, J., Torous, J., Nicholas, J., Carney, R., Rosenbaum, S., Sarris, J. (2017). Can smartphone mental health interventions reduce symptoms of anxiety? A meta-analysis of randomized controlled trials. In *Journal of Affective Disorders*, 218. 10.1016/j.jad.2017.04.046

Fleming, T., Bavin, L., Lucassen, M., Stasiak, K., Hopkins, S., Merry, S. (2018). Beyond the trial: Systematic review of real-world uptake and engagement with digital self-help interventions for depression, low mood, or anxiety. *Journal of Medical Internet Research*, 20(6). 10.2196/jmir.9275

Fonagy, P., Allison, E. (2014). The role of mentalizing and epistemic trust in the therapeutic relationship. *Psychotherapy*, 51(3), 372–380. 10.1037/A0036505

Franco, G.E. (2016). Videogames and therapy: A narrative review of recent publication and application to treatment. *Frontiers in Psychology*, 7, 1085. 10.3389/FPSYG.2016.01085/BIBTEX

Freeman, D., Lister, R., Waite, F., Yu, L. M., Slater, M., Dunn, G., Clark, D. (2019). Automated psychological therapy using virtual reality (VR) for patients with persecutory delusions: Study protocol for a single-blind parallel-group randomised controlled trial (THRIVE). *Trials*, 20(1). 10.1186/s13063-019-3198-6

Furukawa, R., Driessnack, M. (2013). Video-mediated communication to support distant family connectedness. *Clinical Nursing Research*, 22(1), 82–94. 10.1177/1054773812446150

García, E., di Paolo, E.A., de Jaegher, H. (2022). Embodiment in online psychotherapy: A qualitative study. *Psychology and Psychotherapy: Theory, Research and Practice*, 95(1), 191–211. 10.1111/PAPT.12359

Gelso, C.J., Hayes, J.A. (1998). *The Psychotherapy Relationship: Theory, Research, and Practice.* Wiley.

Glucksman, M.L. (2020). The therapeutic relationship reexamined: Clinical and neurobiological aspects of empathic attunement. In *Psychodynamic Psychiatry*, 48(4). 10.1521/pdps.2020.48.4.392

Håland, E., Melby, L. (2015). Negotiating technology-mediated interaction in health care. *Social Theory and Health*, 13(1), 78–98. 10.1057/STH.2014.18/TABLES/1

Han, I., Yang, K.S. (2009). Characteristic analysis for cognition of dangerous driving using automobile black boxes. *International Journal of Automotive Technology*, 10(5). 10.1007/s12239-009-0070-9

Henson, P., Wisniewski, H., Hollis, C., Keshavan, M., Torous, J. (2019). Digital mental health apps and the therapeutic alliance: initial review. *BJPsych Open*, 5(1). 10.1192/bjo.2 018.86

Hooley, J.M., Wilson-Murphy, M. (2012). Adult attachment to transitional objects and borderline personality disorder. *Journal of Personality Disorders*, 26(2). 10.1521/pedi.2012. 26.2.179

Howells, A., Ivtzan, I., Eiroa-Orosa, F.J. (2016). Putting the 'app' in Happiness: A Randomised Controlled Trial of a Smartphone-Based Mindfulness Intervention to Enhance Wellbeing. *Journal of Happiness Studies*, 17(1). 10.1007/s10902-014-9589-1

Huang, H.Y., Bashir, M. (2017). Users' adoption of mental health apps: Examining the impact of information cues. *JMIR MHealth and UHealth*, 5(6). 10.2196/mhealth.6827

Iacoboni, M. (2008). *Mirroring People: The Science of Empathy and How We Connect with Others* (1th ed., p. 316). Farrar, Straus and Giroux. https://books.google.com/books/ about/Mirroring_People.html?hl=pl&id=FEWWzxLlP8YC

Ienca, M., Haselager, P., & Emanuel, E. J. (2018). Brain leaks and consumer neuro-technology. *Nature Biotechnology*, 36(9), 805–810. 10.1038/NBT.4240

Imkamon, T., Saensom, P., Tangamchit, P., Pongpaibool, P. (2008). Detection of hazardous driving behavior using fuzzy logic. *5th International Conference on Electrical Engineering/Electronics*, Computer, Telecommunications and Information Technology, ECTI-CON, 2. 10.1109/ECTICON.2008.4600519

Janzen, J., Fitzpatrick, M., Drapeau, M. (2008). Processes involved in client-nominated relationship building incidents: client attachment, attachment to therapist and session impact. *Psychotherapy*, 45(3), 377–390. 10.1037/A0013310

Jones, E., Lebrun-Harris, L.A., Sripipatana, A., Ngo-Metzger, Q. (2014). Access to mental health services among patients at health centers and factors associated with unmet needs. *Journal of Health Care for the Poor and Underserved*, 25(1). 10.1353/hpu.2014.0056

Keefer, L.A., Landau, M.J., Rothschild, Z.K., Sullivan, D. (2012). Attachment to objects as compensation for close others' perceived unreliability. *Journal of Experimental Social Psychology*, 48(4). 10.1016/j.jesp.2012.02.007

Kim, D.Y., Lee, J.H. (2019). The Effects of Training to Reduce Automatic Action Tendencies Toward Alcohol Using the Virtual Alcohol Approach-Avoidance Task in Heavy Social Drinkers. *Cyberpsychology, Behavior, and Social Networking*, 22(12). 10.1089/ cyber.2019.0121

Kollins, S.H., Childress, A., Heusser, A.C., Lutz, J. (2021). Effectiveness of a digital therapeutic as adjunct to treatment with medication in pediatric ADHD. *Npj Digital Medicine*, 4(1), 1–8. 10.1038/s41746-021-00429-0

Kollins, S.H., DeLoss, D.J., Cañadas, E., Lutz, J., Findling, R.L., Keefe, R.S.E., Epstein, J. N., Cutler, A.J., Faraone, S.V. (2020). A novel digital intervention for actively reducing severity of paediatric ADHD (STARS-ADHD): a randomised controlled trial. *The Lancet Digital Health*, 2(4), 168–178. 10.1016/S2589-7500(20)30017-0/ATTACHMENT/63 DD34AF-B893-4E56-A7A6-2BA8C796C17E/MMC2.MP4

Konok, V., Gigler, D., Bereczky, B.M., Miklósi, Á. (2016). Humans' attachment to their mobile phones and its relationship with interpersonal attachment style. *Computers in Human Behavior*, 61, 537–547. 10.1016/J.CHB.2016.03.062

Koole, S.L., Tschacher, W. (2016). Synchrony in Psychotherapy: A Review and an Integrative Framework for the Therapeutic Alliance. *Frontiers in Psychology*, 7. 10.3389/ FPSYG.2016.00862

Kosinski, M., Bachrach, Y., Kohli, P., Stillwell, D., Graepel, T. (2014). Manifestations of user personality in website choice and behaviour on online social networks. *Machine Learning*, 95(3). 10.1007/s10994-013-5415-y

Krzywinska, T. (2015). Gaming Horror's Horror: Representation, Regulation, and Affect in Survival Horror Videogames. *Journal of Visual Culture*, 14(3). 10.1177/1470412915 607924

Lattie, E.G., Adkins, E.C., Winquist, N., Stiles-Shields, C., Wafford, Q.E., Graham, A.K. (2019a). Digital mental health interventions for depression, anxiety and enhancement of psychological well-being among college students: Systematic review. *Journal of Medical Internet Research*, 21(7). 10.2196/12869

Lattie, E.G., Adkins, E.C., Winquist, N., Stiles-Shields, C., Wafford, Q.E., Graham, A.K. (2019b). Digital mental health interventions for depression, anxiety and enhancement of psychological well-being among college students: Systematic review. *Journal of Medical Internet Research*, 21(7). 10.2196/12869

Leff, J., Williams, G., Huckvale, M.A., Arbuthnot, M., Leff, A.P. (2013). Computer-assisted therapy for medication-resistant auditory hallucinations: Proof-of-concept study. *British Journal of Psychiatry*, 202(6). 10.1192/bjp.bp.112.124883

Levy, K.N., Kivity, Y., Johnson, B.N., Gooch, C. (2018). Adult attachment as a predictor and moderator of psychotherapy outcome: A meta-analysis. *Journal of Clinical Psychology*, 74(11). 10.1002/jclp.22685

Liu, W., Chen, X.J., Wen, Y.T., Winkler, M.H., Paul, P., He, Y.L., Wang, L., Chen, H.X., Li, Y.H. (2020). Memory retrieval-extinction combined with virtual reality reducing drug craving for methamphetamine: Study protocol for a randomized controlled trial. *Frontiers in Psychiatry*, 11. 10.3389/fpsyt.2020.00322

Lombard, M., Ditton, T. (1997). At the heart of it all: The concept of presence. *Journal of Computer-Mediated Communication*, 3(2). 10.1111/J.1083-6101.1997.TB00072.X/4 080403

Luo, S., Jin, J.S., Li, J. (2009). A smart fridge with an ability to enhance health and enable better nutrition. *International Journal of Multimedia and Ubiquitous Engineering*, 4(2).

Mallinckrodt, B. (2010). The psychotherapy relationship as attachment: Evidence and implications. *Journal of Social and Personal Relationships*, 27(2). 10.1177/02654075093 60905

Markowetz, A., Błaszkiewicz, K., Montag, C., Switala, C., Schlaepfer, T.E. (2014). Psycho-Informatics: Big Data shaping modern psychometrics. *Medical Hypotheses*, 82(4). 10.1016/j.mehy.2013.11.030

Marmarosh, C.L., Markin, R.D., Spiegel, E.B. (2013). Attachment in group psychotherapy. In *Attachment in Group Psychotherapy*. American Psychological Association. 10.1037/14186-000

Marshall, J.M., Dunstan, D.A., Bartik, W. (2019a). The Digital Psychiatrist: In Search of Evidence-Based Apps for Anxiety and Depression. In *Frontiers in Psychiatry*, 10. 10.3389/ fpsyt.2019.00831

Marshall, J.M., Dunstan, D.A., Bartik, W. (2019b). The Digital Psychiatrist: In Search of Evidence-Based Apps for Anxiety and Depression. *Frontiers in Psychiatry*, 10, 831. 10.33 89/FPSYT.2019.00831/BIBTEX

Mazri, A., Fiorentini, G. (2017). Light and shadow in online analysis. In J. S. Scharf (Ed.), *Psychoanalysis online* (pp. 65–83).

Mikulincer, M., Shaver, P.R., Berant, E. (2013). An Attachment Perspective on Therapeutic Processes and Outcomes. *Journal of Personality*, 81(6), 606–616. 10.1111/J.14 67-6494.2012.00806.X

Mohr, D.C., Weingardt, K.R., Reddy, M., Schueller, S.M. (2017). Three problems with current digital mental health research. and three things we can do about them. *Psychiatric Services*, 68(5). 10.1176/appi.ps.201600541

Montag, C., Błaszkiewicz, K., Lachmann, B., Sariyska, R., Andone, I., Trendafilov, B., Markowetz, A. (2015). Recorded behavior as a valuable resource for diagnostics in mobile phone addiction: Evidence from psychoinformatics. *Behavioral Sciences*, 5(4). 10.3390/bs5040434

Montag, C., Błaszkiewicz, K., Sariyska, R., Lachmann, B., Andone, I., Trendafilov, B., Eibes, M., Markowetz, A. (2015). Smartphone usage in the 21st century: Who is active on WhatsApp? *BMC Research Notes*, 8(1). 10.1186/s13104-015-1280-z

Myers, E. (1985). Phenomenological Analysis of the Importance of Special Possessions: an Exploratory Study. *Advances in Consumer Research*, 12(1).

Newman, M.G., Szkodny, L.E., Llera, S.J., Przeworski, A. (2011). A review of technology-assisted self-help and minimal contact therapies for anxiety and depression: is human contact necessary for therapeutic efficacy? *Clinical Psychology Review*, 31(1), 89–103. 10. 1016/J.CPR.2010.09.008

Nijman, S.A., Veling, W., Greaves-Lord, K., Vermeer, R.R., Vos, M., Zandee, C.E.R., Zandstra, D.C., Geraets, C.N.W., Pijnenborg, G.H.M. (2019). Dynamic Interactive Social Cognition Training in Virtual Reality (DiSCoVR) for social cognition and social functioning in people with a psychotic disorder: study protocol for a multicenter randomized controlled trial. *BMC Psychiatry*, 19(1). 10.1186/s12888-019-2250-0

Norcross, J.C., Lambert, M.J. (2018). Psychotherapy Relationships That Work III. *Psychotherapy*, 55(4). 10.1037/pst0000193

O'Toole, M.S., Jensen, M.B., Fentz, H.N., Zachariae, R., Hougaard, E. (2014). Emotion differentiation and emotion regulation in high and low socially anxious individuals: An experience-sampling study. *Cognitive Therapy and Research*, 38(4). 10.1007/s10608-014-9611-2

Pericot-Valverde, I., Secades-Villa, R., Gutiérrez-Maldonado, J. (2019). A randomized clinical trial of cue exposure treatment through virtual reality for smoking cessation. *Journal of Substance Abuse Treatment*, 96. 10.1016/j.jsat.2018.10.003

Petrowski, K., Nowacki, K., Pokorny, D., Buchheim, A. (2011). Matching the patient to the therapist: the roles of the attachment status and the helping alliance. *The Journal of Nervous and Mental Disease*, 199(11), 839–844. 10.1097/NMD.0B013E3182349CCE

Porges, S. (2011). *The Polyvagal Theory. Neurophysiological Foundations of Emotions, Attachment, Communication, and Self-regulation*. W. W. Norton.

Pot-Kolder, R.M.C.A., Geraets, C.N.W., Veling, W., van Beilen, M., Staring, A.B.P., Gijsman, H.J., Delespaul, P.A.E.G., van der Gaag, M. (2018). Virtual-reality-based cognitive behavioural therapy versus waiting list control for paranoid ideation and social avoidance in patients with psychotic disorders: a single-blind randomised controlled trial. *The Lancet Psychiatry*, 5(3). 10.1016/S2215-0366(18)30053-1

Qiu, L., Lin, H., Ramsay, J., Yang, F. (2012). You are what you tweet: Personality expression and perception on Twitter. *Journal of Research in Personality*, 46(6). 10.1016/j.jrp.2012.08.008

Rees, C.S., Stone, S. (2005). Therapeutic alliance in face-to-face versus videoconferenced psychotherapy. *Professional Psychology: Research and Practice*, 36(6), 649–653. 10.1037/0735-7028.36.6.649

Riva, G., Teruzzi, T., Anolli, L. (2003). The use of the internet in psychological research: Comparison of online and offline questionnaires. *Cyberpsychology and Behavior*, 6(1). 10.1089/109493103321167983

Romano, V., Janzen, J.I., Fitzpatrick, M.R. (2009). Volunteer client attachment moderates the relationship between trainee therapist attachment and therapist interventions. *Psychotherapy Research*, 19(6). 10.1080/10503300902926547

Rosen, D.C., Nakash, O., Alegría, M. (2016). The impact of computer use on therapeutic alliance and continuance in care during the mental health intake. *Psychotherapy*, 53(1), 117–123. 10.1037/PST0000022

Rus-Calafell, M., Garety, P., Sason, E., Craig, T.J.K., Valmaggia, L.R. (2018). Virtual reality in the assessment and treatment of psychosis: A systematic review of its utility, acceptability and effectiveness. *Psychological Medicine*, 48(3). 10.1017/S0033291717001945

Russell, G.I. (2015). Screen Relations: The Limits of Computer-Mediated Psychoanalysis and Psychotherapy. In *Screen Relations*. Routledge. 10.4324/9780429479762

Sakai, C., Mackie, T.I., Shetgiri, R., Franzen, S., Partap, A., Flores, G., Leslie, L.K. (2014). Mental health beliefs and barriers to accessing mental health services in youth aging out of foster care. *Academic Pediatrics*, 14(6). 10.1016/j.acap.2014.07.003

Schermer, V.L. (2010). Mirror neurons: Their implications for group psychotherapy. *International Journal of Group Psychotherapy*, 60(4). 10.1521/ijgp.2010.60.4.486

Shaw, R. (2004). The embodied psychotherapist: An exploration of the therapists' somatic phenomena within the therapeutic encounter. *Psychotherapy Research*, 14(3), 271–288. 10.1093/PTR/KPH025

Sherman, E. (2019). Reminiscentia: Cherished objects as memorabilia in late-life reminiscence. In *The Meaning of Reminiscence and Life Review*. 10.4324/9781315227269-13

Siegel, D.J. (2019). The mind in psychotherapy: An interpersonal neurobiology framework for understanding and cultivating mental health. *Psychology and Psychotherapy: Theory, Research and Practice*, 92(2), 224–237. 10.1111/PAPT.12228

Simmering, V.R., Ou, L., Bolsinova, M. (2019). What technology can and cannot do to support assessment of non-cognitive skills. *Frontiers in Psychology*, 10(9), 2168. 10.3389/FPSYG.2019.02168/BIBTEX

Slade, A. (2016). Attachment and Adult Psychotherapy: Theory, Research, and Practice. In *Handbook of Attachment. Theory, Research, and Clinical Applications* (3rd ed., pp. 759–779). Guilford Publications.

Torous, J., Firth, J., Huckvale, K., Larsen, M. E., Cosco, T. D., Carney, R., Chan, S., Pratap, A., Yellowlees, P., Wykes, T., Keshavan, M., Christensen, H. (2018). The Emerging Imperative for a Consensus Approach Toward the Rating and Clinical Recommendation of Mental Health Apps. *The Journal of Nervous and Mental Disease*, 206(8). 10.1097/NMD.0000000000000864

Tyrrell, C.L., Dozier, M., Teague, G.B., Fallot, R.D. (1999). Effective treatment relationships for persons with serious psychiatric disorders: the importance of attachment states of mind. *Journal of Consulting and Clinical Psychology*, 67(5), 725–733. 10.1037//0022-006X.67.5.725

Vajawat, B., Varshney, P., Banerjee, D. (2021). Digital Gaming Interventions in Psychiatry: Evidence, Applications and Challenges. *Psychiatry Research*, 295, 113585. 10.1016/J.PSYCHRES.2020.113585

Valmaggia, L.R., Latif, L., Kempton, M.J., Rus-Calafell, M. (2016). Virtual reality in the psychological treatment for mental health problems: An systematic review of recent evidence. *Psychiatry Research*, 236. 10.1016/j.psychres.2016.01.015

Wang, K., Varma, D.S., Prosperi, M. (2018). A systematic review of the effectiveness of mobile apps for monitoring and management of mental health symptoms or disorders. In *Journal of Psychiatric Research*, 107. 10.1016/j.jpsychires.2018.10.006

Wapner, S., Demick, J., Redondo, J.P. (1990). Cherished posessions and adaptation of older people to nursing homes. *International Journal of Aging and Human Development*, 31(3). 10.2190/GJPL-ATJY-KJA3-8C99

Weinberg, H. (2019). Practical considerations for online group therapy. In H. Weinberg & A. Rolnick (Eds.), *Theory and Practice of Online Therapy Internet-delivered Interventions for Individuals, Groups, Families, and Organizations* (1th ed., p. 292). Routledge. 10.4324/9781315545530

Weinberg, H. (2020). Online group psychotherapy: Challenges and possibilities during COVID-19-A practice review. *Group Dynamics*, 24(3), 201–211. 10.1037/GDN0000140

Weinberg, H., Rolnick, A. (2019a). Practical considerations for online individual therapy. In H. Weinberg & A. Rolnick (Eds.), *Theory and Practice of Online Therapy: Internet-delivered Interventions for Individuals, Groups, Families, and Organizations* (1th ed., pp. 96–100). Taylor and Francis. 10.4324/9781315545530-8/PRACTICAL-CONSIDERATIONS-ONLINE-INDIVIDUAL-THERAPY-HAIM-WEINBERG-ARNON-ROLNICK

Weinberg, H., Rolnick, A. (2019b). Introduction. In H. Weinberg & A. Rolnick (Eds.), *Theory and Practice of Online Therapy: Internet-delivered Interventions for Individuals, Groups, Families, and Organizations* (pp. 1–10). Routledge. 10.4324/9781315545530-1

Wexler, A., Reiner, P.B. (2019). Oversight of direct-to-consumer neurotechnologies. *Science*, 363(6424), 234–235. 10.1126/SCIENCE.AAV0223

Winnicott, D. (1953). Transitional objects and transitional phenomena; a study of the first not-me possession. *The International Journal of Psychoanalysis*, 34, 89–97.

Wiseman, R., Watt, C. (2004). Measuring superstitious belief: Why lucky charms matter. *Personality and Individual Differences*, 37(8). 10.1016/j.paid.2004.02.009

Woodhouse, S.S., Schlosser, L.Z., Crook, R.E., Ligiéro, D.P., Gelso, C.J. (2003). Client attachment to therapist: Relations to transference and client recollections of parental caregiving. *Journal of Counseling Psychology*, 50(4), 395–408. 10.1037/0022-0167.50.4.395

Yalom, I., Leszcz, M. (2020). *The Theory and Practice of Group Psychotherapy* (6th ed.). Basic Books. 10.1111/j.1749-6632.1948.tb30971.x

Yarkoni, T. (2012). Psychoinformatics: New Horizons at the Interface of the Psychological and Computing Sciences. *Current Directions in Psychological Science*, 21(6). 10.1177/0963721412457362

Chapter 6

Psychologist dilemmas and challenges in the face of new technologies. Reflections and case studies

E-attachment and clinical practice

Life in a hybrid world is a fact. People have faced globalization that provides new forms of experiences and challenges, especially in relationships. At the time of writing this book, online is as much a part of reality as it is offline – and in fact both are part of everyday life for generations growing up in the 21st century. Clinical practice, both diagnostic and therapeutic, that is transferred to the online reality, and often takes place in a combined way, in the real and virtual world, is not without questions, dilemmas and controversies. Online clinical practice standards have been shaped for several years in various European, Asian and US countries (Chapter 5). However, it is the consequences of the COVID-19 pandemic, including the global lockdown, that confronted clinicians almost all over the world with the need to transfer the diagnostic and therapeutic relationship to an online reality, and consequently to a hybrid reality. The use of new technologies to provide psychological help and to maintain the mental balance of people with emotional difficulties in a crisis has become the method of choice in a pandemic. The presented cases from the authors' own clinical practice are an invitation to reflect on the proverbial basques and shadows of diagnosis and therapy carried out in reality offline-online. The Aurors intention is to invite to a discussion on the conceptualization, techniques, limitations and effectiveness of the process of diagnosis and therapy in hybrid reality, with particular emphasis on the phenomenon of e-attachment[1].

Ania, 11 years old – Individual psychological help

Ania, an 11-year-old patient, showed up at Mental Health Center with her parents, who were concerned about her emotional difficulties. The parents noticed the beginning of the difficulties at the time of the first information about COVID 19. This information came from abroad, but, among other things, prevented the whole family from going abroad for the long-desired winter holiday. So far, the whole family has traveled a lot around the world and spent their time very actively. According to her parents, the girl began to

DOI: 10.4324/9781003221043-7

be fearful and irritable in her parents' opinion; she started to sleep badly. There was reluctance to go to school, which ended many times with staying at home. The girl also began to withdraw from contacts with her peers. Persistent symptoms prompted them to seek help. A child psychiatrist's doctor initially diagnosed Ania with symptoms of depression, although he noted their relationship with stress (Adjustment disorder – 6B43 in ICD 11). Ania did not deny the need to contact a psychologist to whom a psychiatrist referred her. However, she also did not express an open willingness to cooperate with him. She verbally declared that she felt bad, but did not want to develop these threads. At the same time, she did not deny the proposed meetings. She appeared at every meeting and specialists cooperating with her.

The first stage of the therapeutic cooperation with Ania, which continues to this day, started from psychological consultations and diagnosis to the process of psychotherapy. Ania was withdrawn during the meetings, sparing in her statements. She was willing to talk or perform test tasks. However, she resigned, signaling that she was unable to answer the proposed questions or develop a plot. During most of the consultation and diagnostic meetings, she was silent, assuming a tilted, tense body position. It was hard to keep eye contact with her. She looked "frozen", but occasionally also angry. She declared a lack of understanding of the environment (closest and peer) and regret towards others. The drawings hanging in the office, which Ania paid attention to, turned out to be the common space of contact. She commented on them in terms of putting them on the board in the office where the meetings were held. She expressed interest in some of them. She tried to use crayons and cards available next to her spontaneously, but also in a directed manner. Most often, however, she gave up drawing a moment after selecting the crayon, signaling that she did not know what to draw. At that time, we could observe increasing psychomotor tension and withdrawal in Ania. In the declaration of her closest associates, she was distrustful, irritable and unavailable. The time of the pandemic and lockdown influenced the joint decision (of the psychologist, Ania and her parents) to continue online contact.

Psychological online contact in the context of attachment pattern

The 3-month period of regular, weekly online sessions was the time to get to know the world of Ania's inner experiences, establish a diagnostic and therapeutic alliance, define the difficulties, agree and harmonize the goals of further therapeutic contact. At first, online contact with Ania developed through watching Ania's drawings that filled her room, and which the girl from meeting to meeting was more and more willing to present. With time, contact took the form of symbolic communication based on drawing associations about the mood, thoughts and emotions about the meeting itself. Drawings were also a form of intervention that the consulting psychologist decided during this period of time. They concerned impressions, fantasies, associations with what Ania drew and showed for the camera; were a response to her need for symbolic dialogue. They were interventions in the form of reflection, clarification or self-disclosure, with elements of therapeutic play. The drawings of Ania and the consulting psychologist were created during online meetings. Over time, more and more verbal exchanges began to appear around them. Ania became more and more open, she began to explore topics related to the school stress she experienced, experiencing social anxiety from early childhood, ambivalence in relations with her loved ones. She began discussing the experience of alienation and rejection from her early school peers. Her experiences were traumatic; They were overlapped with memories of the loss of people from her closest circle (death/emigration), which the girl experienced in the context of abandonment, regret, and a sense of incomprehension. Often these threads were developed by the girl at the end of the meetings, it was difficult to stop or close them. They were interspersed with sessions full of silence and Neither withdrawal from contact.

What happened in the psychological relationship during this period was changeable, full of tension. Ania's reactions and strategies for coping with tension were inconsistent. Ania ended some sessions in intense, dramatic emotions. Others closing the topic. Sometimes staying withdrawn and at a distance. The analysis of Ania's way of experiencing, her perception of the environment and reactions during subsequent online sessions indicated that the girl's development was based on an unorganized pattern of attachment. She was accompanied by a high level of anxiety and avoidance. On the one hand, the online contact forced by the pandemic and its consequences was conducive to lowering Ania's anxiety and establishing a psychological alliance. It allowed for a greater understanding of the girl's inner experiences, an initial conceptualization of her problems and the goals of further therapeutic help. However, it is difficult to verify how much impact the online itself had in this regard, and to what extent it was the effect of the duration of the contact and its repeatability. The ability to connect from home, from your own room seemed to be conducive to Ania's sense of security. On the other hand, especially in situations of intense emotional reaction, the question arose of how to effectively contain them. The possibilities in this area have decreased, and certainly changed when switching to online contact. The symbolic ritual of leaving another space, of returning home, has disappeared. Time has been reformulated. Ending the session was embedded in turning off the camera and closing the laptop hatch. Working on developing a ritual that would give the opportunity for emotional closure after the session ended turned out to be crucial during the 3 months of online contact.

Online contact ended with the easing of restrictions and the possibility of returning face-to-face contact. Ania ended it with more openness and a declaration about the need for psychotherapeutic work. At the end of the process of psychological help described above, the experience of common ground, relationship, emerged. Ania ended this stage knowing and understanding what the proposed psychotherapy is. The ability to control anxiety, tension and frustration emerged enough to persevere in a helping relationship. The girl started psychotherapeutic contact in direct contact.

Laura, 40 years old- Individual psychotherapy

Laura, a 40-year-old patient, came to the Mental Health Center with symptoms of persistent pessimism in the patient's thinking, low self-esteem, lack of self-confidence, symptoms of apathy, persistent low mood, difficulty falling asleep, nightmares, perceived constant fatigue and anxiety. After consulting a psychiatrist, she received a diagnosis of depression-anxiety disorders (the equivalent of Mixed depressive and anxiety disorder – 6A73 in ICD 11). The onset of symptoms appeared after the birth of the third daughter, three years before reporting to a psychiatrist. Until she came to psychotherapy, she was treated with pharmacotherapy, with no visible effects.

By the age of 40, symptoms of depression and anxiety had increased greatly. The need for perfectionism that emerged as a consequence of persistent symptoms or the desire to be well assessed and present at the best possible side has become extremely tiring. In contact with the psychologist, she presented herself as insecure, silent, difficult to establish verbal contact. Laura was proposed individual psychotherapy in the psychodynamic current.

The first stage of 12-month-long (meetings once a week) of individual psychotherapy was carried out in face-to-face contact. This stage was focused on building a therapeutic alliance and clarifying how Ms. Laura defines her problem (the feeling of being unable to function effectively as a mother and as a professional doctor, and the associated sense of failure). In the course of the psychotherapeutic process, Laura began to explore her life threads, tell her life story, reflecting on the connection of childhood experiences and patterns of thinking formed at that time (especially in relationships with relatives, her caregivers and other people) with the current, anxious-depressive pattern of relationships with other people.

During the 12 months of meetings, Laura initially canceled the sessions, explaining that she did not look after the children. However, there was a gradual building of confidence in the therapist. Laura herself noticed that she is more open, she learns to talk about herself and her emotions – although she has never done it before. Nevertheless, her psychotherapy was interrupted by single absences. The anxiety-depressive symptoms (including nightmares) persisted. During the individual contact in direct contact, the psychotherapist did not have the feeling that the moment when it was possible to talk about emotional insight had been reached. Due to the state of the pandemic and its consequences in the form of a lockdown, Laura was referred to online individual psychotherapy in order to maintain the psychotherapeutic process, which she agreed to.

Online psychotherapy in the context of attachment pattern

During the 24-month online therapy, Laura gradually gained cognitive and then emotional insight into learning about internal attachment patterns, formed in childhood and their relationship with her current anxious and depressive experience of contacts with other people. The analysis of Laura's way of experiencing and her behavior in relations with the outside environment (family, husband and social environment) indicated that she exhibited an attachment style characterized by high attachment anxiety, and high attachment avoidance. One could observe in her relationships, experiencing and behaving a high level of anxiety, excessive perfectionism and obsessiveness as well as a sense of alienation, "being on the side", a tendency to avoid relationships with others. Laura showed a great deal of distrust towards others and a depressiveness that was growing alongside anxiety. It oscillated between approaching and avoiding.

During the online session, the patient did not cancel the session, she came to them regularly, discussing systematically experienced mental well-being, coping with everyday difficulties in social relations (including partner relations), pointing more and more boldly and clearly on the range of different emotions felt in relation to the social environment. She began to explore topics related to: closeness with caregivers, the experience of the anxiety pattern of experiencing adolescence, alienation in contacts with peers, fear of relationships, blocked experiencing adolescent rebellion. She analyzed the background of the nightmares experienced from childhood to still nightmares, clarified the patterns of emotional closeness with partners (suppressing anger, fear of confrontation), and internal conflicts related to the marriage relationship. She also began discussing the topic of the relationship with the therapist. She suggested that online psychotherapy allows her to be more open. She began to analyze her anxiety in a therapeutic relationship, anger, helplessness, and at the same time emotions experienced in the role of a mother (anxiety, anger, exhaustion, helplessness, but also joy, love, closeness). She also linked the theme of her own child's puberty to her own maturation. An important thread during online meetings, which did not appear during face-to-face meetings, was the thread of anger and hatred as well as assertiveness in expressing emotions. At the end of the online psychotherapeutic process, a common experience of alliance, relationship, and the sense of security declared by Laura appeared in the therapy process.

Symptomatic improvement appeared, followed by the need to go on vacation and return to professional development. After returning to the sessions, the threads of positive emotions related to the joy and willingness to "act" began to appear at the sessions. The topic of ending the therapy appeared and the therapist reacted approvingly. He expressed his interest in the stage of a noticeable change in the reduction of anxiety symptoms and pessimistic thinking. He reacted with an intervention that encouraged him to experiment with new, assertive behaviors. At the end of the online contact with Laura, she stated that she was ready to end the therapy in order to achieve her goals (the ability to recognize and express emotions, greater self-awareness, self-acceptance, the ability to ask for help).

Laura directly referred to online contact, claiming that she could participate in it more often and that this form was more acceptable to her. This can be understood as a signal that online psychotherapy (de facto forced by the pandemic process) made it possible to find a certain zone of psychological comfort; reduction of anxiety and tension enough to stop fiddling with it. Consequently, it was possible to form a real alliance based on trust.

The decision to end online therapy in this case was not tantamount to achieving all therapeutic goals. Nevertheless, there was a permanent symptomatic improvement, which allowed Laura to return to professional activities and feel life satisfaction and psychophysical well-being.

Online psychodynamicgrouppsychotherapy

Online group psychotherapy, although known and practiced for many years, has not yet received as much empirical research as online individual psychotherapy. In the literature, we can find reports of support groups, or mindfulness or yoga groups, or CBT groups (Weinberg, 2020; Bantjes et al., 2021). Basically, there is less research on groups based on emotions and relationships (psychodynamic, interpersonal approach) (Kocijan et al., 2021; Jesser et al., 2021).

The four women described below participated in an online psychodynamic group psychotherapy for ten weeks, in setting twice a week for 2 one-hour sessions[2]. The choice of these people for description is not accidental – each of the participants of the described psychotherapy obtained a different result in the Experience in Close Relationship questionnaires, so each had a slightly different attachment characteristic. For the sake of secrecy and structuring the data presented, these women are presented here as:

- Mrs A with secure attachment style,
- Mrs B with preoccupied attachment style,
- Mrs C with avoident attachment style,
- Mrs D with secure attachment style.

The table below (Table 6.1) presents the basic characteristics and issues of the described women, taking into account the dimensions and styles of the relationship.

The shortened issue of the indicated women corresponds with the attachment style, in the form of a specific way of building relationships with others or regulating affect. The analysis presented below focuses on two selected aspects:

1   building relationships with the group during the on-line therapy. Measurement points were made in 1, 4, 7 and 10 – the last week of therapy;
2   the effects of therapy according to the pre-post-follow up methodology, i.e. measurements were made in the 1st and 10th week of therapy and 6 weeks after its completion. Details are presented in the drawings and tables.

Table 6.1 The basic characteristics and issues of the described women, taking into account the dimensions and styles of the relationship

X	Axiety dimension (fear of abandonment and rejection)	
Avoidance dimension (fear of closeness and discomfort with dependence on others)	**Secure** (low anxiety, low avoidance) Mrs A, 45, married, works, has not participated in psychotherapy before. Reported problems: due to mobbing at work, he has fears and a depressed mood, wakes up at night, cries, has stomach pains. Psychiatric diagnosis according to ICD-11: Adjustment disorder – 6B43	**Preoccupied** (high anxiety, low avoidance) Mrs B, 24, in a partnership with a man but lives with his parents, works. She had previously participated in individual psychotherapy. Reported problems: two crisis situations – the mother fell ill with oncology and broke up with her boyfriend and entered into a new, complicated relationship. Great fear of being left alone, crying, depressed mood, difficulty concentrating, body symptoms: trembling hands and body tremors. You have had thoughts of suicide in the past. Psychiatric diagnosis according to ICD-11: Adjustment disorder – 6B43
	Avoidance (low anxiety, high avoidance) Mrs C, 30, miss, works, lives alone, previously participated in individual psychotherapy. Reported problems: psychosomatic symptoms, mainly from the digestive system, high level of perceived stress. Difficulties in relationships – he relates, but later cannot keep. She decided to live alone. Psychiatric diagnosis according to ICD-11: Bodily distress disorder – 6C20; suspected personality disorder	**Fearful** (high anxiety, high avoidance) Mrs D, 60, after divorce, retired, lives alone, many years ago she participated in therapy for women after domestic violence, which she stopped. Problems reported: difficulty coping with overwhelming emotions, bouts of anger and aggression alternating with depression. In the interview, a long history of trauma, in the family of origin and in relationships in adulthood. One suicide attempt in the past. Psychiatric diagnosis according to ICD-11: Personality disorder – 6D10 (In ICD 10: F60.9 Mixed personality disorder, respectively)

COHESION TO GROUP

Mrs A. (Secure)   Mrs B. (Preoccupied)   Mrs C. (Avoidant)   Mrs D. (Fearful)

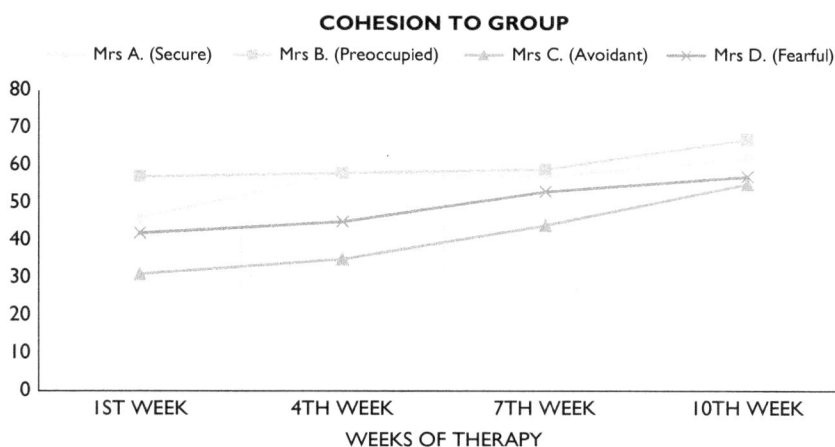

Figure 6.1 The online group psychotherapy-cohesion of the group.

Cohesion of the group

In group psychotherapy, group cohesion is treated as an equivalent of the therapeutic relationship. The research used a tool to study the perception of relationships with a group – The Group Experience Questionnaire by J. Eckert and B. Strauß (Wiergiles et al., 2011). Coherence was defined in this questionnaire as feeling satisfied with being in a group. Figure 6.1 below shows the dynamics of changes in terms of the sense of cohesion with the group for each of the four women discussed.

The chart above shows that at the beginning of online group therapy, Mrs B (Preoccupied Attachment Style) and Mrs A (Secure Attachment Style) showed the greatest coherence with the group. People with preoccupied attachment style show the greatest need for close bonds with others and strive to build close relationships as soon as possible, fearing loneliness. This probably explains the highest result in the first week. In turn, the lowest score was obtained by Mrs C (Avoidant Attachment Style), which can also be understood in the context of the dynamics of this attachment style, where the attachment system is deactivated and relational feelings are "cooled".

There are also some facts worth paying attention to. Until the end, Mrs B held her highest group consistency score. Mrs C had the lowest score until the very end. Mrs A had a mean consistency score at the beginning, consistency increased in the first 4 weeks and remained at a similar, stable level throughout. In all women, an increase in the declared level of cohesion with the group was observed over time. This can be understood as a signal that a relationship has been built and that group cohesion has been formed in the process of online group psychotherapy. It is worth recalling here that group cohesion is considered to be one of the most important therapeutic factors in group psychotherapy.

Hostility to the group and therapist

Another variable studied by The Group Experience Questionnaire is Hostility to the group and therapist. Figure 6.2 shows what dynamics of hostility characterized the described women with different attachment styles.

It was observed that the highest level of hostility towards the group and the therapist was presented by Mrs B (Preoccupied Attachment Style), i.e. the same person who, at the same time, in the first week of therapy presented the highest level of perceived consistency with the group (Figure 6.1). Preoccupied attachment style is the counterpart of the axious–ambivalent pattern of attachment seen in children, characterized by conflicting feelings: clinging to the caregiver without regulating emotions, showing resistance and hostility at the same time. Probably such a phenomenon also took place here. Ultimately, people with insecure attachment styles (Mrs B, Mrs C and Mrs D) had a similar score at week 10. Mrs A (Secure attachment Style) showed a low level of hostility, which even decreased during the therapy. It can also be noticed that in Mrs C (Avoidant attachment Styles) as the only one, the level of hostility increased during the therapy. It can be understood that with the growing cohesion with the group, but also the probable fear of closeness, the balancing (cooling) mechanism in the form of hostility also had to be activated.

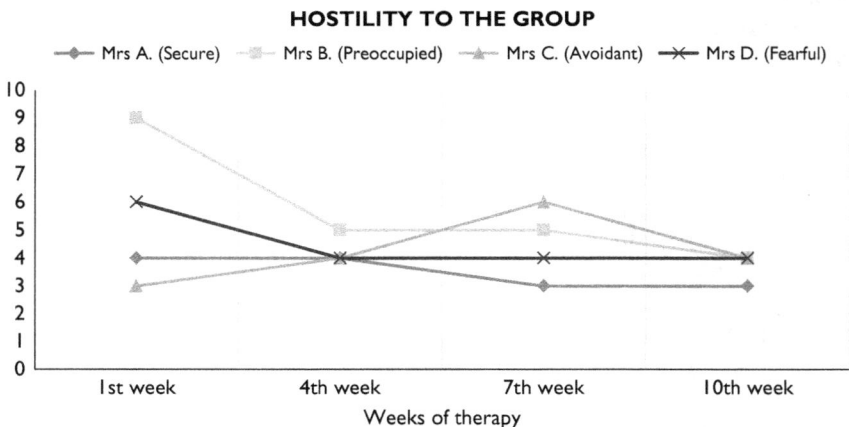

Figure 6.2 The online group psychotherapy-hostility to the group.

LACK OF COURAGE IN EXPRESSING ONESELF

Figure: Line chart. Legend: Mrs A. (Secure), Mrs B. (Preoccupied), Mrs C. (Avoidant), Mrs D. (Fearful). Y-axis 0 to 20. X-axis: 1ST WEEK, 4TH WEEK, 7TH WEEK, 10TH WEEK. Axis label: WEEKS OF THERAPY.

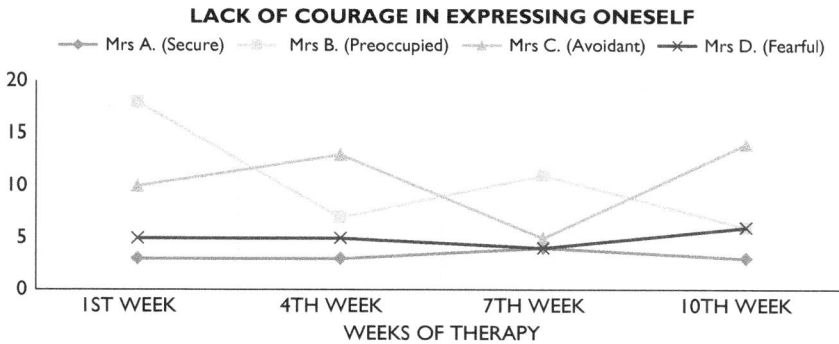

Figure 6.3 The online group psychotherapy-lack of courage in expressing oneself.

Lack of Courage in expressing oneself

Another variable in the group process tested with The Group Experience Questionnaire is Lack of courage in self-expression. Figure 6.3 presents the dynamics of patients in this respect.

Mrs A (Secure Attachment Styles), of the four of them, seemed to have a stable ability to express themselves courageously. It is worth noting, however, that Mrs C's (Avoidant Attachment Style) lack of courage in self-expression grew during the therapy, briefly decreasing in the 7th week. Interestingly, it was also associated with an increased feeling of hostility (Figure 6.2). It can be assumed that in week 7 Mrs C developed more courage in self-expression and thus hostility. The authors leave to the readers reflection why it happened in this period of time.

Unsatisfied waiting for help

The last examined variable of the group process was the unsatisfied expectation of help felt by the women presented. Figure 6.4 shows the dynamics of this variable.

The lowest level of unsatisfied expectation of help is seen in Mrs C (Avoidant Attachment Style), which can probably be explained by the low level of needs directed towards others. On the other hand, for Mrs B and Mrs D Unsatisfied expectation of help is high. It is difficult to determine whether it is related to the characteristics of the patients themselves (attachment style) or whether the nature of the therapy should also be taken into account (that online therapy was unsatisfactory for them). It can be imagined that such patients, with an increased need to strive for others in a remote relationship, felt too little closeness and thus showed a high level of unsatisfied expectation of help. This is one of the hypotheses. Aspects related to the formal effects of therapy could be equally important here.

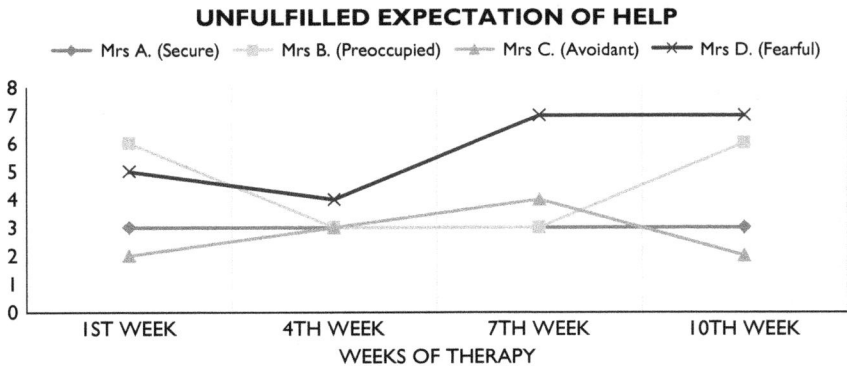

Figure 6.4 The online group psychotherapy-unfulfilled expectation of help.

Therapy effects

The effects of therapy in the described project were measured, inter alia, by the shortened Polish version of the Symptom Checklist (SCL–27pl) (.....), where the positive effect was understood as the reduction of symptoms. SCL–27pl allows to establish the Global Severity Index and 5 subscales: depressive symptoms, vegetative symptoms, symptoms of social phobia, symptoms of agoraphobia and pain symptoms. In this description, for the sake of clarity, only the Global Severity Index has been presented. Another variable showing change in online group therapy was self-esteem, as measured by the Rosenberg Self-Esteem Scale (SES). Here, a positive result was understood as an increase in self-esteem.

The tables below present the results from the 1st week of therapy (pretest), from the 10th week of therapy (post-test) and the results from the 6th week after the end of the therapy (follow-up). In addition to the result obtained, the difference for the posttest-pretest and follow-up-poesttes results is also shown. The Reliable Change Index (RCI) was also calculated for the difference from the last and the end week of therapy. RCI computed by dividing the difference between the pretreatment and posttreatment scores by the standard error of the difference between the two scores, and the RCI value ≥1.96 is interpreted as significant. This result can be regarded as a real change at the clinical level (Table 6.2).

It was observed that the overall symptom level decreased at the end of online therapy in Mrs A., Mrs B., Mrs C., with the RCI index showing that probably only a significant change had occurred in Mrs A with secure attachment style. In case of Mrs. D with fearful attachment, there was an increase in symptoms which probably indicates a deterioration in therapy but without a significant RCI. Interestingly, 6 weeks after the end of the therapy, her general symptom score decreased significantly.

Table 6.2 Changes in the general level of neurotic symptoms during group psychotherapy in 4 women with different attachment styles

Participants	Global Severity Index SCL-27PL				
	1st week	*10th week*	*Difference post-pretreatment*	*Follow-up 6th week after therapy*	*Difference follow-up – posttreatment*
Mrs A. (Secure)	24	5	−19 (RCI = 2.82)[*]	17	12
Mrs B. (Preoccupied)	21	9	−12 (RCI = 1.78)	19	10
Mrs C. (Avoidant)	48	45	−3 (RCI = 0.44)	43	−2
Mrs D. (Fearful)	31	39	8 (RCI = 1.19)	23	−16

Note
* RCI ≥1.96; SCL-27PL–Symptom Checklist.

Table 6.3 shows that in all people there was an increase in self-esteem, and the RCI index suggests that in as many as three people it is a clinically significant increase: in Mrs A, Mrs B. and Mrs D. In Mrs A. the increase in self-esteem is also progressing 6 weeks after the end of psychotherapy, while Mrs C's self-esteem decreased after the therapy. Taking into account these selective data, it can be argued that the secure attachment style Mrs A clearly benefited from online group therapy. In the case of other people, it is difficult to talk about "taking advantage" of the online psychotherapy process in a group form.

These observations are compatible with the personal declarations of the presented participants, for which they were asked at the end of psychotherapy. The exact question asked in the questionnaire was: "Please, give free comment, free thoughts (optional question)". All people decided to enter a comment in the space provided. The Table 6.4 presents the comments of the four described women.

Table 6.3 Changes in self-esteem during group psychotherapy in patients with different attachment styles

Participants	Rosenberg Self-Esteem Scale				
	1th week	*10th week*	*Difference post-pretreatment*	*Follow-up 6th week after therapy*	*Difference follow-up – posttreatment*
Mrs A. (Secure)	23	29	6 (RCI = 2.45)[*]	35	6
Mrs B. (Preoccupied)	18	24	6 (RCI = 2.45)[*]	24	0
Mrs C. (Avoidant)	17	20	3 (RCI = 1.23)	16	−4
Mrs D. (Fearful)	22	31	9 (RCI = 3.68)[*]	32	1

Note
* RCI ≥1.96; SCL-27PL– Symptom Checklist.

Table 6.4 Opinions about on online psychotherapy according to the described participants

X	Anxiety dimension (fear of abandonment and rejection)
Avoidance dimension (fear of closeness and discomfort with dependence on others)	**Secure** (low anxiety, low avoidance) <u>Mrs A:</u> a convenient form of therapy as it is given from home. The therapy not only fulfilled my goals, but also showed me many other things that I would like to deal with. However, I very much regret that you cannot keep in touch with other participants of the therapy. So far, on-line psychotherapy has been a better form of therapy for me than the previous one. * Due to the number of treatments per week. The therapy twice a week allowed me to better see my emotions and behavior. **Avoidance** (low anxiety, high avoidance) <u>Mrs C:</u> it was the first time that I participated in group psychotherapy. I was full of fear that I would not find myself and that the difficulty of working in a group, which I have always had, would multiply. I was afraid that I would not speak, because I would find that what I have to say is of little importance, and indeed it was so at many moments. But there were also times when I broke through and that is a great achievement for me. The most pleasant thing, however, was that my weakest moments were always noticed by someone from the group and dragged me into the conversation. It made me feel part of the group and felt that I was important to someone. I felt taken care of by the rest. The only disappointment for me is that the whole therapy is so short and I feel internal disappointment, sadness and fear that it is over. In retrospect, I also think that I would prefer the therapist to be more frequent and give us more feedback. **Preoccupied** (high anxiety, low avoidance) <u>Mrs B:</u> the therapist was very professional. Psychotherapy met my expectations, I would like to start a new group psychotherapy. **Fearful** (high anxiety, high avoidance) <u>Mrs D:</u> a huge plus is that you do not notice any negative reactions in the participant, i.e. excessive sweating of the hands, shaking hands caused by emotions, changes in the color of the face, these are embarrassing symptoms. Nevertheless, a conversation with a "living" person face to face is a great value, because you can interact smoothly. Openness, learning to control overly violent emotions, unrelated to the adequacy of such emotions, talking and not closing in and sealing negative emotions.

Note
* The patient had not participated in psychotherapy before, only in a few regular, individual meetings of a diagnostic and counseling nature in a private psychological office.

What draws attention is the fact that the longest written statement, appreciating the therapy and regretting that it was too short, was presented by Mrs C, a person with avoidant attachment style. This is the same person who declared the lowest level of cohesion with the group among those analyzed here, and did not experience any change in symptoms and self-esteem. Probably the online form gave the opportunity to interact with people without a significant "threat of closeness and bond", not without significance is also the fact that the statement was in writing under the Nick used in the research process (i.e. anonymously and impersonally). Probably the opposite was the case with Mrs B who left a very laconic description, which could be interpreted as a lack of "interest in contact with the form". Perhaps she was more interested in real contact with the person, and not in the task of filling out a form. Mrs D, in turn, pointed out that the advantage of online psychotherapy lies in the ability to conceal difficulties in controlling affect and the associated physiological responses.

Searching for an answer

Online diagnostic and psychotherapeutic contact has become a fact in the era of a pandemic. Even if it was treated as a transitional one at the time of writing this book, it has ceased to be. It makes it possible to implement this aid where it has not been possible so far. Also in those places where direct contact becomes a real threat to security. The rapidly developing forms of online psychological help, psychotherapy and clinical diagnosis with the use of advanced technologies open up a number of questions. They include setting, structure, technical issues, as well as boundaries, security, space for making independent and independent decisions. These are the questions that guide the ethical search for the future.

Notes

1 The term e-attachment was introduced and defined by the authors in Chapter 2 of this monograph.
2 One of the authors of this book has conducted a research project (2021-2022) on the effectiveness and other aspects of online group psychodynamic psychotherapy. The study involved 22 participants, distributed in two groups conducted online in the psychodynamic paradigm. The therapy was scheduled twice a week, with 2 one-hour sessions of group psychotherapy, thus it included 40 therapeutic sessions over 10 weeks.

References

Bantjes, J., Kazdin, A.E., Cuijpers, P., Breet, E., Dunn-Coetzee, M., Davids, C., Stein, D.J., Kessler, R.C. (2021). A Web-Based Group Cognitive Behavioral Therapy Intervention for Symptoms of Anxiety and Depression Among University Students: Open-Label, Pragmatic Trial. *JMIR Mental Health*, 8(5), e27400. DOI: 10.2196/27400

Jesser, A., Muckenhuber, J., Lunglmayr, B., Dale, R., Humer, E. (2021).Provision of Psychodynamic Psychotherapy in Austria during the COVID-19 Pandemic: A Cross-Sectional Study. *International Journal of Environmental Research and Public Health*, 18(17), 9046. DOI: 10.3390/ijerph18179046

Kocijan, L.S., Caratan, S., Ivrlač, A., Gorišić, L., Šimunović Filipčić, I., Filipčić, I. (2021). How to Square a Circle? *PsychiatriaDanubina*, 33(4), 702–705. PMID: 34718306.

Weinberg, H. (2020). Online Group Psychotherapy: Challenges and Possibilities During COVID-19—A Practice Review. *Group Dynamics: Theory, Research, and Practice*, 24(3), 201–211. DOI: 10.1037/gdn0000140

Wiergiles, J., Janke-Klimaszewska B. i Tomczak, K. (2011). Adaptacja polskiej wersji Kwestionariusza Doświadczenia Grupowego J. Eckerta i B. Straussa do badania procesów zachodzących w grupie terapeutycznej. *Psychoterapia*, 3(158), 61–70.

Chapter 7

Summing up

The issue of online contact in the area of diagnosis and therapy is currently the subject of research interest. The change brought about by the development of information and communication technology (ICT), in retrospect, can be safely called a breakthrough. The expansion of tools for remote communication, Portable Electronic Devices (PEDs) and the hybrid way of functioning of today's generations have put psychologists, psychotherapists and clinicians in front of new challenges. The discussion on "whether" to introduce online communication into the process of psychological diagnosis and the sphere of psychological help and psychotherapy was changed into a discussion of "how". The key issue in this discussion is the issue of attachment as a construct necessary to shape the basic sense of security and psychological comfort of a human being. It seems that the well-established view, despite the civilization and technological breakthrough, is the perception of the significant role of attachment in shaping the psychological development path of a given person, but its significant importance for the nature of interpersonal relations, including the diagnostic and therapeutic relationship. However, it seems a mistake to assume a priori that the existing paradigms regarding the formation of a pattern, and then the attachment style in direct contact, can be transferred to an understanding of how attachment is formed in a hybrid reality. This is especially true of those generations that experience contact and exchange from conception through virtual reality, not just physical contact.

The COVID-19 pandemic has undoubtedly forced an even greater focus on the topic of introducing digital technology to diagnostic and therapeutic procedures. Completion of this monograph coincided with the lecture of the authors, at the national conference of clinical psychology, on research and practical attempts to introduce into the virtual world the equivalents of bonds, social touch, physical and emotional presence of others. The successive appearance of applications, methods and devices to support the building of relationships and attachment bonds in the connected offline space – online reopens topics already discussed in diagnosis and therapy. Each of the authors of this monograph has encountered the situation of looking for a convenient place to talk online, technical problems with connecting at the climax of the

DOI: 10.4324/9781003221043-8

session or uncontrolled access to information from the private life, sometimes intimate of the patient. Thus, he gained access to information that would be disclosed in direct contact, if at all, rather in a gradual manner, with the development and duration of the diagnostic and therapeutic alliance. Apart from a series of questions about setting, boundaries and ethics, it also poses the need for participants of such a professional relationship to change their communication habits. Psychologists, clinicians and therapists are also faced with the need to adapt the adopted models of conceptualization and work to the changing reality. What's more, also adaptation to the emerging sense of intrusive entering the world of another person or changing the content to be contained in the process of diagnosis and therapy.

Are these considerations exaggerated? Is it justified to use the notion of E-attachment even in a working sense? Is it not an overinterpretation in relation to the already well-described phenomenon of attachment, currently realizing itself in a digital reality changed by an aspect of technology? When looking for answers to these questions, one can refer to the famous thought experiment about consciousness (Mary's room) by professor Frank Jackson. It concerns the image of a scientist with specialist knowledge of neurophysiology and human perception of color. At the same time, the idea that she lives in a black and white world is therefore deprived of the perceptual experience of color. One day, Mary leaves the room and notices red for the first time. Will Mary's knowledge so far prove sufficient? Will it change (will gain new knowledge) as a result of this experience?

A hybrid way of functioning, online communication, transferring development, relations and the basis for shaping attachment to the digital network becomes a fact. Is it good or bad, according to a Chinese proverb, we will see. The answer to these dilemmas may, however, be the assumption that an e-attachment could exist. The very assumption of such a possibility seems to be developing and creative in the attitude towards the clinical and, at the same time, scientific understanding of interpersonal relations and psychological phenomena in contemporary reality.

Index

For Product Safety Concerns and Information please contact our EU
representative GPSR@taylorandfrancis.com
Taylor & Francis Verlag GmbH, Kaufingerstraße 24, 80331 München, Germany